ABC of
Mental

Second Edition

ABC series

An outstanding collection of resources - written by specialists for non-specialists

The *ABC series* contains a wealth of indispensable resources for GPs, GP registrars, junior doctors, doctors in training and all those in primary care

- **Now fully revised and updated**

- **Highly illustrated, informative and practical source of knowledge**

- **An easy-to-use resource, covering the symptoms, investigations, treatment and management of conditions presenting in your day-to-day practice and patient support**

- **Full colour photographs and illustrations aid diagnosis and patient understanding of a condition**

For more information on all books in the *ABC series*, including links to further information, references and links to the latest official guidelines, please visit:

www.abcbookseries.com

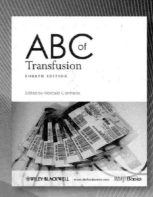

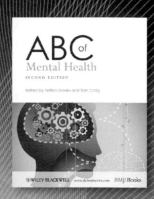

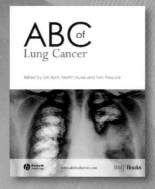

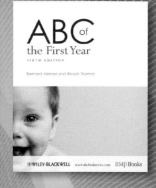

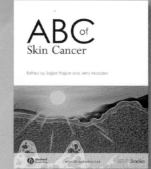

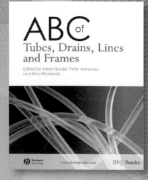

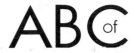

ABC of

Mental Health

Second Edition

EDITED BY

Teifion Davies
Senior Lecturer in Community Psychiatry
King's College London Institute of Psychiatry
London, UK

Tom Craig
Professor
Section of Social Psychiatry
King's College London Institute of Psychiatry
London, UK

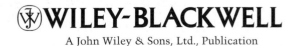

WILEY-BLACKWELL
A John Wiley & Sons, Ltd., Publication

BMJ|Books

This edition first published 2009, © 1998, 2009 by Blackwell Publishing Ltd

BMJ Books is an imprint of BMJ Publishing Group Limited, used under licence by Blackwell Publishing which was acquired by John Wiley & Sons in February 2007. Blackwell's publishing programme has been merged with Wiley's global Scientific, Technical and Medical business to form Wiley-Blackwell.

Registered office: John Wiley & Sons Ltd, The Atrium, Southern Gate, Chichester, West Sussex, PO19 8SQ, UK

Editorial offices: 9600 Garsington Road, Oxford, OX4 2DQ, UK
The Atrium, Southern Gate, Chichester, West Sussex, PO19 8SQ, UK
111 River Street, Hoboken, NJ 07030-5774, USA

For details of our global editorial offices, for customer services and for information about how to apply for permission to reuse the copyright material in this book please see our website at www.wiley.com/wiley-blackwell

Library of Congress Cataloging-in-Publication Data

ABC of mental health / [edited by] Teifion Davies, Tom Craig. -- 2nd ed.
   p. ; cm.
   Includes bibliographical references and index.
   ISBN 978-0-7279-1639-6 (alk. paper)
   1. Mental health services--Handbooks, manuals, etc. I. Davies, Teifion. II. Craig, T. K. J. (Thomas K. J.)
   [DNLM: 1. Mental Disorders. 2. Community Mental Health Services. WM 140 A134 2008]

   RA790.5.A225 2008
   616'89--dc22

                                                          2008006130

ISBN: 978-0-7279-1639-6

A catalogue record for this book is available from the British Library.

Set in 9.25/12 pt Minion by Newgen Imaging Systems (P) Ltd, Chennai, India
Printed & bound in Singapore by Ho Printing Singapore Pte Ltd

2   2010

Contents

Contributors, vii

Preface, ix

List of Abbreviations, x

1 Mental Health Assessment, 1
Teifion Davies and Tom Craig

2 Managing Distressed and Challenging Patients, 7
Teifion Davies

3 Mental Health Problems in Primary Care, 11
Richard Byng and Jed Boardman

4 Managing Mental Health Problems in the General Hospital, 15
Amanda Ramirez and Allan House

5 Mental Health Emergencies, 19
Zerrin Atakan and David Taylor

6 Mental Health Services, 23
Rosalind Ramsay and Frank Holloway

7 Anxiety, 28
Stirling Moorey and Anthony S Hale

8 Depression, 35
Anthony S Hale and Teifion Davies

9 Bipolar Disorders, 40
Teifion Davies

10 Schizophrenia, 44
Trevor Turner

11 Disorders of Personality, 48
Martin Marlowe

12 Psychosexual Problems, 52
Dinesh Bhugra, James P Watson and Teifion Davies

13 Addiction and Dependence: Illicit Drugs, 55
Clare Gerada and Mark Ashworth

14 Addiction and Dependence: Alcohol, 60
Mark Ashworth, Clare Gerada and Yvonne Doyle

15 Mental Health Problems in Old Age, 64
Chris Ball

Contents

16 Dementia, 68
Chris Ball

17 Mental Health Problems of Children and Adolescents, 72
Emily Simonoff

18 Mental Health Problems in People with Intellectual Disability, 76
Nick Bouras and Geraldine Holt

19 Mental Health in a Multiethnic Society, 81
Simon Dein

20 Mental Health on the Margins: Homelessness and Mental Disorder, 86
Philip Timms and Adrian McLachlan

21 Mental Health and the Law, 91
Humphrey Needham-Bennett

22 Drug Treatments in Mental Health, 96
Soumitra R Pathare and Carol Paton

23 Psychological Treatments, 103
Suzanne Jolley and Phil Richardson

24 Risk Management in Mental Health, 108
Teifion Davies

Index, 114

Contributors

Mark Ashworth
General Practitioner
Hurley Clinic, Lambeth
London, UK

Zerrin Atakan
Consultant Psychiatrist
South London and Maudsley NHS Foundation Trust
London, UK

Chris Ball
Consultant Psychiatrist in Mental Health of Older Adults
South London and Maudsley NHS Foundation Trust
London, UK

Dinesh Bhugra
Professor of Mental Health and Cultural Diversity
King's College London Institute of Psychiatry
London, UK

Jed Boardman
Senior Lecturer in Social Psychiatry
Health Services Research Department
King's College London Institute of Psychiatry
London, UK

Nick Bouras
Professor of Psychiatry
Estia Centre
King's College London Institute of Psychiatry
London, UK

Richard Byng
GP and Senior Clinical Research Fellow
Peninsula Medical School
Plymouth, UK

Tom Craig
Professor
Section of Social Psychiatry
King's College London Institute of Psychiatry
London, UK

Teifion Davies
Senior Lecturer in Community Psychiatry
King's College London Institute of Psychiatry
London, UK

Simon Dein
Senior Lecturer
Centre for Behavioural and Social Sciences in Medicine
University College London
London, UK

Yvonne Doyle
Regional Director of Public Health
NHS South East Coast
Horley, UK

Clare Gerada
Director, RCGP Substance Misuse Unit
Hurley Clinic, Lambeth
London, UK

Anthony S Hale
Professor of Psychiatry
Kent Institute of Medicine and Health Sciences
University of Kent
Canterbury, UK

Frank Holloway
Consultant Psychiatrist
South London and Maudsley NHS Foundation Trust
London, UK

Geraldine Holt
Consultant Psychiatrist
Estia Centre
King's College London Institute of Psychiatry
London, UK

Allan House
Professor of Liaison Psychiatry
University of Leeds
Leeds, UK

Suzanne Jolley
Research Clinical Psychologist
King's College London Institute of Psychiatry
London, UK

Martin Marlowe
Consultant Psychiatrist
Bath North CMHT, Bath NHS Trust
Bath, UK

Adrian McLachlan

General Practitioner
Hetherington Practice, Clapham
London, UK

Stirling Moorey

Consultant Psychiatrist
South London and Maudsley NHS Foundation Trust
London, UK

Humphrey Needham-Bennett

Consultant Forensic Psychiatrist & Caldicott Guardian
South London and Maudsley NHS Foundation Trust
London, UK

Soumitra R Pathare

Consultant Psychiatrist
Ruby Hall Clinic
Pune, India

Carol Paton

Chief Pharmacist
Oxleas NHS Foundation Trust
Dartford, UK

Amanda Ramirez

Professor and Director
Cancer Research UK London Psychosocial Group
King's College London Institute of Psychiatry
London, UK

Rosalind Ramsay

Consultant Psychiatrist
South London and Maudsley NHS Foundation Trust
London, UK

Phil Richardson

(Deceased)
Professor of Clinical Psychology
University of Essex
Colchester, UK

Emily Simonoff

Professor of Child and Adolescent Psychiatry
King's College London Institute of Psychiatry
London, UK

David Taylor

Chief Pharmacist
South London and Maudsley NHS Foundation Trust
London, UK

Philip Timms

Consultant Psychiatrist
START Team
South London and Maudsley NHS Foundation Trust
London, UK

Trevor Turner

Consultant Psychiatrist
East London and The City Mental Health NHS Trust
London, UK

James P Watson

Formerly Professor of Psychiatry
United Medical and Dental Schools
London, UK

Preface

Mental health problems are among the most common reasons that patients consult doctors, and many of these consultations take place in primary care, in the accident and emergency department, or in the outpatient clinics and wards of the general hospital. Indeed, the high prevalence of mental health problems means that all health-care professionals and many social care and educational professionals will encounter people experiencing mental health problems, so all clinicians require basic mental health skills. The *ABC of Mental Health* gives all clinicians guidance on practical management of mental disorders in an easily accessible format. It provides essential information needed to recognise and manage significant mental disorders safely and successfully, from detecting symptoms, through choice of treatments, to decisions about when and how to seek specialist advice.

There have been many significant changes in the 10 years since the publication of the first edition of the *ABC of Mental Health*. Although the disorders seen by clinicians have changed little, the range of treatments available and the guidelines for their use have changed greatly. Newer psychotropic drugs have replaced typical antipsychotics and tricyclic antidepressants in the first-line treatment of schizophrenia and depression, and already concerns have emerged about their unwanted effects (metabolic syndrome with the atypical antipsychotics; suicidality with some antidepressants). Guidance from the National Institute for Health and Clinical Excellence (NICE) has systematised treatment regimens, and emphasised the efficacy of psychological treatments such as cognitive behavioural therapy (CBT) for several disorders.

In the UK, the organisation of mental health services (including the care programme approach) has evolved, and new legislation has amended the framework within which these services operate (Human Rights Act 1998; Mental Capacity Act 2005; Mental Health Act 2007). Within mental health services, there has been an increased emphasis on risk assessment. Populations at risk have changed too, with the numbers of people from ethnic minority backgrounds up 50% in 10 years. This edition of the *ABC of Mental Health* takes account of these and other changes.

The book begins with an introduction to assessment of a patient's mental health problems, and then deals with the disorders most frequently encountered in particular settings, such as primary care and the general hospital. The major categories of mental disorder are covered next in greater detail, followed by chapters on the main mental health needs of vulnerable groups (elderly people, children, ethnic minorities, homeless people). The final chapters cover broader issues of management: guidance on medication and psychological treatments, the law, and risk management.

Managing mental health problems is a multidisciplinary task. We hope that the book will appeal not only to doctors, but to members of all professions involved in mental health: nursing, social work, counselling, and the law (both lawyers and police). We believe its accessibility will encourage debate, the use of a common language between professionals, and, ultimately, better management of people with mental health problems.

We are indebted to two anonymous referees and we are sure they will recognise their suggestions and comments in these chapters. We thank Adam Gilbert and Helen Harvey of Wiley-Blackwell for their patience and perseverance over many months.

Teifion Davies
Tom Craig

List of Abbreviations

ACE	angiotensin converting enzyme		GGT	gamma-glutamyl transferase
ACI	acetylcholinesterase inhibitors		GHS	General Household Survey
ACT	acceptance and commitment therapy		GMC	General Medical Council
AD	Alzheimer type dementia		GMS	General Medical Services
ADHD	attention deficit hyperactivity disorder		HIV	human immunodeficiency virus
AIDS	acquired immunodeficiency syndrome		HTT	home treatment team
AMHP	approved mental health professional		ICD	International Classification of Disease
AMTS	Abbreviated Mental Test Score		ID	intellectual disability
AOT	assertive outreach team		IPT	interpersonal therapy
ASW	approved social worker		LBD	Lewy body dementia
AUDIT	Alcohol Use Disorders Identification Test		LFT	liver function test
BME	black and ethnic minority		MAPPA	multi-agency public protection arrangements
BMI	body mass index		MAOI	monoamine oxidase inhibitors
CAF	Common Assessment Framework		MCV	mean corpuscular volume
CAMHS	child and adolescent mental health services		MDO	mentally disordered offenders
CAT	cognitive analytic therapy		MMSE	Mini-Mental State Examination
CBT	cognitive behavioural therapy		MRI	magnetic resonance imaging
CIAMHS	Croydon Integrated Adult Mental Health Service		MST	multisystems therapy
CMHT	community mental health team		NHS	National Health Service
CPA	Care Programme Approach		NICE	National Institute for Health and Clinical Excellence
CPN	community psychiatric nurse		NSAID	nonsteroidal anti-inflammatory drug
CRT	crisis resolution team		NSF	National Service Framework
CSM	Committee on Safety of Medicines		OCD	obsessive–compulsive disorder
CT	computed tomography		PDD	pervasive developmental disorder
CTO	community treatment order		PTSD	post-traumatic stress disorder
DBT	dialectical behaviour therapy		RC	responsible clinician
DSM	Diagnostical and Statistical Manual		RMO	responsible medical officer
DUP	duration of untreated psychosis		RT	rapid tranquillisation
ECG	electrocardiogram		SIB	self-injurious behaviours
EEG	electroencephalogram		SMR	standardised mortality ratio
EIT	early intervention team		SNRI	selective serotonin-noradrenaline reuptake inhibitor
EMDR	eye movement desensitisation reprocessing		SOAD	second opinion approved doctors
EMG	electromyelogram		SSRI	selective serotonin reuptake inhibitor
EPSE	extrapyramidal side effects		TCA	tricyclic antidepressant
FBC	full blood count		TFT	thyroid function test
FI	family intervention		U & Es	urea and electrolytes
GABA	gamma-aminobutyric acid		VD	vascular dementia
GAD	generalised anxiety disorder		VDRL	venereal disease research laboratory test

CHAPTER 1

Mental Health Assessment

Teifion Davies and Tom Craig

OVERVIEW

- Mental health problems affect about a third of the adult population at any time, and all clinicians should be familiar with their recognition and initial assessment

- Mental health or psychiatric assessment follows a similar pattern to assessment in other clinical specialities: history of the presenting complaint, formal examination, investigation and diagnosis

- A full picture of the patient's problems may be built up over several interviews, and broadened to include collateral history from family and friends

- An initial interview with a distressed patient has important therapeutic value

Psychiatry in healthcare

Symptoms of mental disorder are common: at any time, about a third of the adult population reports suffering from distressing symptoms such as worry, sleep disturbance or irritability. According to the World Health Organization, mental disorders comprise five of the top 10 causes of years lived with disability, accounting for about 22% of the total disability worldwide. All healthcare professionals will encounter people experiencing mental health problems, so all clinicians require basic mental health skills (Box 1.1).

Psychiatry is the branch of medicine that deals with disorders in which mental (emotional or cognitive) or behavioural features are most prominent. The cause, presentation and course of such disorders are influenced by diverse factors; their symptoms can be bewildering to patients and their relatives; and their management may require social and psychological as well as medical interventions. It is not surprising that this complex situation can lead to misunderstandings regarding the role of psychiatrists (who are neither social workers nor gaolers) and myths about the practice of psychiatry.

The bulk of mild mental disorders has always been managed by family doctors. Patients referred to psychiatrists are increasingly likely to be managed at home by community mental health services or, if admitted to an acute psychiatric ward, to be discharged after

Box 1.1 **Prevalence of psychiatric morbidity**

- **Mental symptoms:** 30% of adults experience worry, tension, irritability or sleep disturbance at any time
- **All mental disorders:** >20% of adults at any time suffer mental health problems; 25% of general practice consultations involve mental health problems
- **Depression (including mixed anxiety and depression):** 10% of adults depressed in a week; 55% depressed at some time
- **Anxiety disorders:** >10% of adults have clinically important symptoms (about 5% generalised anxiety, 5–10% phobias, 1% each for obsessive–compulsive disorder, post-traumatic stress disorder and panic disorder)
- **Suicide:** rate in UK falling (now 8/100,000 per year) but rising elsewhere; 4000 deaths and more than 100,000 attempts annually; 5% of all years of life lost in people aged under 75 years
- **Self-harm:** 1 in 600 people harm themselves sufficiently to require hospital admission; 1% of these go on to kill themselves
- **Schizophrenia (and other functional psychoses):** 0.4% of people living at home; 1% lifetime risk; 10 patients on a typical general practice list, but 10,000 not registered with a general practitioner
- **Bipolar affective disorder:** at least 2% of adults
- **Personality disorder:** 5–10% of young adults
- **Alcohol-related disorder:** 4.7% of adults show alcohol dependence
- **Drug dependence:** 2.2% of adults living at home
- **Anorexia nervosa:** 1% of adolescent girls

a short stay. Many former long-stay patients have been discharged to the community with varying degrees of support and supervision. This book will deal with the principles and practice of managing mental health problems.

Psychiatric assessment

There is a myth that psychiatric assessment differs from that in other medical specialties: it does not, it follows the familiar sequence of history, examination (both mental state and physical) and investigation, leading to differential diagnosis. Another myth holds that management cannot proceed without obtaining an extensive history that delves into all aspects of a patient's life. Diagnosis can take only a few minutes, but time must be spent fleshing out

ABC of Mental Health, 2nd edition. Edited by T. Davies and T. Craig.
©2009 Blackwell Publishing, ISBN: 978-0-7279-1639-6.

the initial impressions, assessing immediate risks and collecting information about personal and social circumstances that modify symptoms or affect management and long-term prognosis.

Accuracy is achieved by close attention to the pattern of evolution of presenting symptoms and examination of a patient's mental state. A complete psychiatric assessment requires a detailed personal history, which, if the doctor is not familiar with the patient, may be built up over a series of interviews. The important point is that such detail comes into play only once the basic problem has been ascertained clearly.

Good interview technique

Interview technique is important in all branches of medicine. A good psychiatric interview comprises a series of 'nested' processes of gathering information in which gathering of general information is followed by specific questions to clarify ambiguities and confirm or refute initial impressions (Boxes 1.2 and 1.3).

Open questions

The interview begins with open questions concerning the nature of the present problem, followed by more focused questions to clarify chronological sequences and the evolution of key symptoms. Open questions encourage patients to talk about matters of immediate concern to them and help to establish a rapport.

Closed questions

Specific closed questions (equivalent to the systematic inquiry of general medicine) should follow only when a clear outline of the underlying disorder has emerged. These questions form a checklist of symptoms often found in variants of the likely disorder but not mentioned spontaneously by the patient (such as diurnal variation of mood in severe depression).

Box 1.2 **Examples of useful open and closed questions**

Open questions
- Is anything troubling you?
- Could you say a little more about it/them?
- And …?
- Is there anything else you want to mention (worrying you)?
- Tell me about your daily routine (your family, your upbringing)
- Are there any questions you want to ask me?

Closed questions
- When did these problems (thoughts, feelings) begin?
- How do they affect you (your life, your family, your job)?
- Have you experienced anything like this in the past?
- What do you think caused these problems?
- What exactly do you mean when you say you feel depressed (paranoid, you can't cope)?
- At times like these, do you think of killing yourself?
- Do you hear voices (or see images) when nobody seems to be there?

Choice questions
- Is it like …, or like …, or like something else?

Box 1.3 **Dos and don'ts in the psychiatric interview**

Do
- Do let the patient tell his or her story
- Do take the patient seriously
- Do allow time for emotions to calm
- Do inquire about thoughts of suicide or violence
- Do offer reassurance where possible
- Do start to forge a trusting relationship
- Do remember that listening is doing something

Don't
- Don't use closed questions too soon
- Don't pay more attention to the case notes than to the patient
- Don't be too rigid or disorganised: exert flexible control
- Don't avoid sensitive topics (such as ideas of harm to self or others) or embarrassing ones (such as sexual history)
- Don't take at face value technical words the patient might use (such as depressed, paranoid)

Remember
- Put your patient at ease – it is an interview not an interrogation
- Be neutral – avoid pressure to 'take sides' or to collude with or against the patient

---

Choice questions

Sometimes patients are not accustomed to answering open questions. This is often so with adolescents and children, who are more used to being told how they feel by adults. In these cases, a choice question may be more useful. This suggests a range of possible answers to the patient but always allows for replies outside the suggested range: 'Do you feel like …, or …, or something else?'

On each topic the interview should move smoothly from open questions to more closed, focused questions

---

Initial assessment

The first and most important stage entails getting a clear account of current problems (presenting complaint and mental state), social circumstances and an estimate of concurrent physical illness (including substance misuse) that might influence the presentation.

Once the current situation is clear and rapport has been established, closed questions should be used to elicit specific items of history. Topics covered at this stage include patient's prior psychiatric and medical problems (and their treatment), use of alcohol and prescribed and illicit drugs, and level of functioning at home and at work. Initial suspicions of risk to the patient or others should be clarified gently but thoroughly.

Risk assessment

It is a myth that asking about suicidal ideas may lead patients to consider suicide for the first time. Fleeting thoughts of suicide are common in people with mental health problems. Importantly, intensely suicidal thoughts can be frightening, and sufferers are often relieved to find someone to whom they can be revealed.

Persecutory beliefs, especially those focusing on specific people, should be elicited clearly as they are associated with dangerousness. Patients who ask for complete confidentiality – 'Promise you won't tell anyone' – should be reassured sympathetically but firmly that the duty to respect their confidence can be overridden only by the duty to protect their own or others' safety.

Assessment of capacity

All patients must be assumed to have the capacity to make decisions for themselves about their care and treatment. Where there is doubt about this capacity, it must be assessed formally according to the Mental Capacity Act: this will be covered in more detail in Chapter 21.

Mental state examination

Whereas the history relates to events and experiences up to the present time, the mental state examination focuses on current symptoms and signs using closed questions. This bears direct analogy to the physical examination and is an attempt to elicit, in an objective way, the signs of mental disorder. The emphasis is now on the form as well as the content of the responses to well-defined questions covering a range of mental phenomena. For example, the form of a patient's thought may be delusional, and the content of the delusions may concern abnormal beliefs about family or neighbours (Box 1.4).

Physical examination and investigation

Relevant physical examination is an important part of the assessment and should follow as soon as is practicable. Usually, this will require only simple cardiovascular (pulse, blood pressure) and neurological (muscle tone and reflexes, cranial nerves) examination. Similarly, laboratory investigations (Box 1.5) should be performed

---

Box 1.5 **Tests and investigations**

- **Primary level:** full blood count (including red cell morphology); electrolytes; liver function tests; ECG; urine drug screen; breath alcohol
- **Secondary level:** chest X-ray; skull X-ray; renal function (e.g. creatinine clearance); blood chemistry (e.g. calcium, glucose, HbA_{1c}, thyroid function, drug levels, B_{12}, iron); serology (e.g. syphilis, hepatitis, HIV)
- **Tertiary level:** EEG; sleep EEG; CT and MR imaging; EMG

This approach clarifies the choice of psychiatric investigations
- Primary level tests should be considered for every patient and if not performed, the reasons for omission should be recorded
- Secondary and tertiary level tests should be performed only if indicated by the presentation, by other findings or on specialist advice, and the reasons for their performance recorded

---

as indicated, considering a patient's past health and intended treatment. The choice may be influenced by

- Patient's age
- Known or suspected concurrent physical disease
- Alcohol or substance misuse
- Intended drug treatment (e.g. antidepressants, antipsychotics or lithium). An electrocardiogram should be considered before starting drugs with known cardiac effects, and body mass index (BMI) calculated before starting treatment with drugs that affect metabolism
- Concurrent medication (several drugs potentiate the cardiac effects of antidepressants and antipsychotics).

Further inquiry

The second broad phase of assessment involves gathering information to place the present complaint in the context of a patient's psychosocial development, premorbid personality and current circumstances. This phase also follows the scheme of open and then closed questioning, but, because of the breadth of the issues to be covered, it is often the longest component of a psychiatric assessment. Whenever possible, a collateral history should be obtained from those who know the patient (family, friends or carers).

Box 1.4 **Important items of mental state examination**

- **Appearance:** attire, cleanliness; posture and gait
- **Behaviour:** facial expression; cooperation or aggression; activity, agitation, level of arousal (including physiological signs)
- **Speech:** form and pattern; volume and rate; is it coherent, logical and congruent with questioning?
- **Mood:** apathetic, irritable, labile; optimistic or pessimistic; thoughts of suicide; do reported experience and observable mood agree?
- **Thought:** particular preoccupations; ideas and beliefs; are they rational, fixed or delusional? Do they concern the safety of the patient or other people?
- **Perception:** abnormalities including hallucinations occurring in any modality (auditory, visual, smell, taste, touch)
- **Intellect:** brief note of cognitive and intellectual function; is the patient orientated in time, place and person? Is the patient able to function intellectually at a level expected from his or her history?
- **Insight:** how does the patient explain or attribute his or her symptoms?

For a disturbed patient who is bewildered by his or her bizarre experiences, the interview may be a critical period and the doctor should not waste it

---

Much of this information may not be available initially, or may take too long to collect in a busy surgery or accident and emergency department. There is no reason to delay urgent management while this information is sought. Similarly, sensitive issues such as a patient's psychosexual history should not be avoided but can be elicited more easily when the patient's trust has been gained.

Therapeutic importance of the psychiatric interview

The interview is more than an information gathering process: it is the first stage of active management. This may be the first opportunity for a patient to tell his or her full story or to be taken seriously, and the experience should be beneficial in itself. The length of the interview should allow time for intense emotions to calm and for the first steps to be taken towards a trusting therapeutic relationship. The balance between information gathering and therapeutic aspects of the interview is easily lost if, say, a doctor works relentlessly through a pre-set questionnaire or checklist of symptoms.

Making sense of psychiatric symptoms

Although psychiatric symptoms can be clearly bizarre, many are recognisable as part of normal experience. The situation is identical to the assessment of pain: a doctor cannot experience a patient's pain nor measure it objectively but is still able to assess its significance. A pattern can be built up by comparing the patient's reported pain – its intensity, quality and localisation – with observation of the patient's behaviour and any disability associated with it. Similarly, patients' complaints of 'feeling depressed' may be linked to specific events in their life, to a pervasive sense of low self-esteem, or to somatic features such as disturbed sleep and diurnal variation in mood.

Another myth is that the vagueness of psychiatric features makes diagnosis impossible (Box 1.6). In fact, psychiatric diagnoses based on current classification systems are highly reliable. It is true that

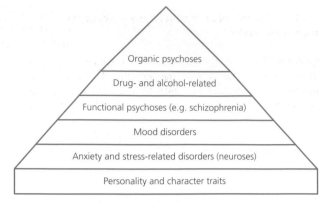

Figure 1.1 Diagnostic hierarchy of psychiatric disorders
- Each level *includes* all symptoms of all lower levels. A disorder may show any of the features of disorders below it at some time, but these are not characteristic of that disorder
- Each level *excludes* symptoms typical of higher levels
- In patients with a higher level disorder (such as schizophrenia) it may be important to treat 'lower level' symptoms (such as depression)
- A patient's enduring personality and character traits will modify his or her presentation of symptoms to healthcare services
- Coexisting physical disease and treatment will affect, and be affected by, the presentation of mental disorder.

there are no pathognomonic signs in psychiatry – that is, most psychiatric signs in isolation have low predictive validity, as similar features may occur in several different disorders. It is the pattern of symptoms and signs that is paramount.

In practice, sense may be made of the relation between features and disorders by envisaging a hierarchy in which the organic disorders are at the top, the psychoses and neuroses in the middle, and personality traits at the bottom (Figure 1.1). A disorder is likely to show the features of any of those below it in the hierarchy at some time during its course but is unlikely to show features of a disorder above it. Thus, a diagnosis of schizophrenia depends on the presence of specific delusions and hallucinations and will often include symptoms of anxiety, depressed mood or obsessional ideas; it is much less likely if consciousness is impaired (characteristic of delirium, which is higher in the hierarchy). Conversely, personality factors will influence the presentation of all mental (and physical) disorders as they are at the foot of the hierarchy.

Summarising the findings

A bare diagnosis rarely does justice to the complexity of a presentation, nor does it provide an adequate guide to management. The formulation is a succinct summary of a patient's history, current circumstances and main problems: it aims to set the diagnosis in context. It is particularly useful in conveying essential information, as when making a referral to specialist psychiatric services (Box 1.7). An adequate referral to such services should include
- Description of the presenting complaint, its intensity and duration
- Relevant current and past medical history and medication
- Findings of mental state examination
- Physical health and any drug treatment

Box 1.6 **Some troublesome terms used in psychiatry**

- **Psychosis** is best viewed as a process in which the patient's experience and reasoning do not reflect reality. Psychotic symptoms (hallucinations and delusions) may occur transiently in several physical and mental disorders and are not pathognomonic of any disorder. Psychotic disorders are ones that are characterised by psychotic symptoms
- **Neurosis** is a portmanteau term for disorders in which anxiety or emotional symptoms are prominent. It is falling from use as it is difficult to define, has been applied too broadly, and gives no guide to aetiology, intensity or course
- **Delusion** is a false belief held with absolute conviction and not amenable to argument (incorrigible) or to explanation in terms of the patient's culture. It may be bizarre, but this is not necessarily so
- **Hallucination** is a false perception arising without an external stimulus: it is experienced as real and vivid, and occurring in external space (that is, 'outside' the patient's head). In contrast, an illusion is a misinterpretation of a real external stimulus
- **Confusion** is a mild and transient state, in which there is fluctuation in level of consciousness, with impairment of attention and memory
- **Delirium** implies a more severe impairment of consciousness, usually of organic origin, with hallucinations and delusions

---

Organic psychoses
Drug- and alcohol-related
Functional psychoses (e.g. schizophrenia)
Mood disorders
Anxiety and stress-related disorders (neuroses)
Personality and character traits

- Estimate of degree of urgency in terms of risk to the patient and others
- Indication of referrer's expectations (assessment, advice, admission)
- Very urgent requests may be brief but should be reinforced by telephone.

Consequences of mental disorder

Patients with mental disorders often suffer *stigma* – the experience of being discriminated against and rejected by others, and a consequent feeling of shame and disgrace. There may also be other serious consequences.

Mortality rates

Psychiatric disorders are associated with increased risk of death from all causes, and the all-cause standardised mortality ratio (SMR) among community psychiatric patients is about 1.6 (that is, about 1.6 times the rate in the general population). Mortality rates are highest among people suffering schizophrenia (SMR 1.76), men (SMR 2.24), and younger patients (SMR 8.82 for ages 14 to 24 years). So-called avoidable deaths are four times higher in patients with psychiatric diagnoses than in the general population. Some of this excess is due to suicide and violence, some to higher rates of respiratory, cardiac, and other diseases, and some to lack of appropriate healthcare. In some surveys, over 50% of patients smoked more than 15 cigarettes per day.

Disability rates

The World Health Organization estimates mental disorders to have a disproportionate effect on disability worldwide: mood disorders, schizophrenia and alcohol misuse cause about 20% of the days lived with disability. Depression alone contributes almost 5% of the global burden of disease, is worse in women and in developing countries, and reduces recovery from a range of physical illnesses.

Fitness to drive

A driver with a mental disorder has a slightly increased risk of being involved in a road traffic accident, with personality disorders, alcohol intoxication, and side effects of drug treatment accounting for most of the increase. Some disorders (such as schizophrenia, bipolar affective disorder) affect a driver's entitlement to hold a driving licence, at least during the acute illness and for 6–12 months afterwards. For other disorders, the period of withdrawal of the licence will depend on the severity of the condition, and may be permanent in some cases (such as severe dementia). Patients have a duty to inform the licensing authority of any such disorder, and the doctor should do this where a patient is unable or unwilling to do so. Care should be taken to warn patients of potential side effects of drug treatment that might affect their driving.

Other aspects

Suffering from mental disorder might affect life insurance premiums, while being detained under the Mental Health Act may restrict a patient's voting rights. Local guidance should be sought in cases of doubt.

Role of voluntary organisations

Several local and national voluntary organisations are concerned with mental health. They may provide telephone advice or support, counselling, day centres, and volunteers or befriending services. Many patients benefit from the counselling or mutual support offered by such organisations, self-help groups and charities. These include patients with severe or protracted mental disorders and their carers, and many others who are distressed by unpleasant circumstances but are not suffering from a mental disorder and so do not require a referral to specialist mental health services.

Further information

The following organisations produce useful leaflets on various aspects of mental health
- Royal College of Psychiatrists, 17 Belgrave Square, London SW1X 8PG www.rcpsych.ac.uk/mentalhealthinformation.aspx
- The Mental Health Foundation www.mentalhealth.org.uk/information/mental-health-a-z/
- MIND www.mind.org.uk/Information/
- Rethink (National Schizophrenia Fellowship) www.rethink.org/about_mental_illness/index.html

Personal accounts of mental health problems

Hopley M. *Metronome*. Chipmunkapublishing, Brentwood, Essex, 2005. www.chipmunka.com

Kennedy VJ. *Mad In England*. Chipmunkapublishing, Brentwood, Essex, 2007. www.chipmunka.com

Knight S. *Black Magic*. Chipmunkapublishing, Brentwood, Essex, 2007. www.chipmunka.com

Wealthall K. *Little Steps*. Chipmunkapublishing, Brentwood, Essex, 2005. www.chipmunka.com

Further reading

Davies T. Psychiatric symptoms. In: Rees J and Gibson T, eds. *Essential clinical medicine*. Cambridge University Press, Cambridge, 2009.

DVLA Drivers Medical Group. *At a glance guide to the current medical standards of fitness to drive.* www.dvla.gov.uk/medical/ataglance.aspx

Mathers CD, Loncar D. Projections of global mortality and burden of disease from 2002 to 2030. *PLoS Med* 2006; **3**: e442. doi:10. 1371/journal. pmed.0030442

National Institute for Health and Clinical Excellence. *Mental health and behavioural conditions.* NICE, London, http://guidance.nice.org.uk/topic/behavioural

Poole R, Higgo R. *Psychiatric interviewing and assessment.* Cambridge University Press, Cambridge, 2006.

Semple D *et al. Oxford handbook of psychiatry.* Oxford University Press, Oxford, 2005.

CHAPTER 2

Managing Distressed and Challenging Patients

Teifion Davies

OVERVIEW

- A minority of patients have dysfunctional coping abilities that may cause difficulties for them and the clinicians they consult
- Managing emotional distress is very similar to managing the distress and desperation experienced by the patient in severe pain
- A clinician should be able to recognise, acknowledge, contain and reflect the patient's distress
- The key to satisfactory management is negotiating and agreeing achievable goals for both patient and clinician

Box 2.1 **Coping patterns**

Functional	Dysfunctional
Multi-faceted	Pervasive
Wide ranging	Limited
Flexible	Inflexible, stereotyped
Adaptable	Maladaptive
Modifiable	Unmodifiable

Most people with health problems – mental or physical – present only clinical challenges to their doctors and others who care for them. However, a small proportion of patients present a challenge due to their behaviour, and when this is associated with longstanding mental health problems, especially personality problems, the impact on the doctor–patient relationship can be significant. In one survey, physicians rated about 15% of their patients (and 25% of those with mental health problems) as 'difficult'; and suggested that those with particular symptoms (abdominal pain, headache, insomnia) were most likely to pose non-clinical challenges. A UK Healthcare Commission survey found that about a third of NHS staff encounter abuse or violence each year.

Coping patterns

Mental and physical health problems can both contribute to and result from a patient's experience of stressful circumstances. When faced with a frightening or distressing situation, people react generally in line with coping strategies they have learned during their early development and modified with later experience (Box 2.1). In any individual, functional patterns of coping will vary slightly depending on circumstances, be broadly in proportion to the type and intensity of stress, and change over time in line with experience.

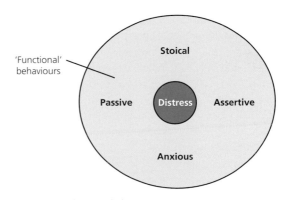

Figure 2.1 Functional coping behaviours.

However, if the magnitude of the stress is overwhelming the response will be less flexible and more stereotyped. In some cases, the threshold at which the individual's coping strategies are overwhelmed is very low, with the result that he or she will react in a stereotyped and disproportionate manner to apparently minor upset. Also, for some, the ability to learn from experience is limited or biased so that coping tends to become more rather than less dysfunctional with time.

Coping and behaviour

As individuals exhibit varying degrees of effectiveness in coping with stressful or distressing circumstances, their coping will be reflected in their behaviours. Some typical examples of functional coping behaviours are shown in Figure 2.1. So, the patient who is coping functionally with distress may exhibit a variety of responses at different times: sometimes stoical, but at others worrying and

ABC of Mental Health, 2nd edition. Edited by T. Davies and T. Craig. ©2009 Blackwell Publishing, ISBN: 978-0-7279-1639-6.

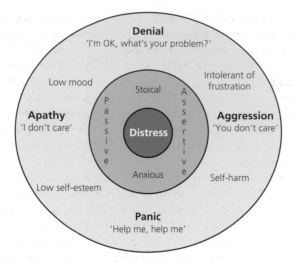

Figure 2.2 Dysfunctional coping behaviours.

anxious; mixing passive acceptance of fate with an acceptable degree of assertiveness or determination. In general, he or she will exhibit behaviours that are adapted to and modified by the specific context, and so may behave differently towards his or her family, clinicians, or friends and acquaintances. Multi-faceted behaviours are characteristic of normal coping.

When the individual's ability to cope with distress is overwhelmed, his or her pattern becomes both exaggerated and fixed (Figure 2.2). Stoicism becomes frank denial, assertiveness merges into outright aggression, and so on. More importantly, the multi-faceted behaviours are lost and a pervasive, inflexible pattern emerges that is similar in all circumstances. So family, friends, clinicians and strangers are all met with the same disproportionate display.

Just as behaviours viewed favourably (patience, resilience, cooperation, adherence) will produce a positive response from clinicians, so behaviours viewed unfavourably (impatience, complaining, anger, non-compliance) will elicit a negative response; in either case, the effect of each encounter is to reinforce and amplify the patient's behavioural responses to similar situations. Where a patient might have ongoing distressing symptoms, the cumulative effect of many such encounters – each one relatively minor – is to sensitise the patient to any hint of disapproval or rejection from clinicians, especially doctors.

Managing difficult behaviours

While the most serious behavioural disturbances, involving physical violence or damage to property, might require exceptional measures (police or security staff, removal from a practice list), many can be contained and managed by the use of a set of techniques with which all clinicians will be familiar and use routinely as part of everyday clinical practice (Box 2.2). Thus, the aim is not so much to extend the clinician's repertoire of skills as to apply those that are already of use in other, less threatening, clinical situations.

Pain management model

A first step in managing the difficult patient is to have a conceptual framework or model within which to make sense of the patient's behaviour. Every clinician is familiar with the distress caused by pain, and the desperation that a patient might experience when suffering intense pain from a potentially life-threatening disorder. In such circumstances, a patient's behaviour, although unacceptable in other contexts, might be viewed benignly and met with understanding and reassurance. The crucial advantage of recognising the analogy with pain, and applying a pain management model, is that the clinician feels competent and confident to manage the crisis (Box 2.3). All other steps in managing a patient's distress, and any unacceptable behaviour, stem from this recognition.

Recognising behavioural expressions of distress

Most doctors and other clinicians will be familiar with unacceptable verbal expressions of a patient's distress. Some common examples are listed in Box 2.4. Each of these themes may be delivered with varying degrees of annoyance, anger, abuse or even aggression.

Box 2.2 General principles of managing distress

- Conceptualise emotional distress as similar to pain
- Recognise the behavioural expressions of distress
- Acknowledge distress in similar manner to acknowledgment of pain
- Contain distress
- Reflect the expression of distress back to patient
- Model appropriate behaviours
- Outline – and agree – achievable goals

Box 2.3 Steps to understanding distress – analogy with pain

- Emotional distress is similar to the distress caused by pain
- It may be acute and frightening, or chronic and debilitating, or both
- Behaviour is an expression of this distress, confirmed and amplified by:
  - Lack of previous positive experience of healthcare
  - Little confidence, or trust, in professional competence
  - Expectation of rejection
  - Sensitivity to negative reactions

Box 2.4 Verbal expressions of distress

Frustration	• It's now or never
	• If I don't get help now, it will be too late
	• You just don't want to help me
Rejection	• You pretend to care
	• You don't like me
	• If you send me away …
Undermining	• I thought doctors were supposed to help
	• You aren't able to help me
	• If you won't help me …
	• You're useless
Threatening	• You'll regret this
	• You made me do it
	• They will blame you
	• It's all your fault

Clearly, it is important to recognise the mannerisms associated with escalating tension. Although these are generally well known, it is too easy to overlook them in a busy consultation. A patient may remain standing, or rise from the chair, during the interview and pace about the room. He or she may avoid eye contact, or stare at the clinician or into space; volume, tone and speed of speaking may change, becoming loud or very quiet, rapid or slow and emphatic. His or her posture may change, becoming tense and rigid, or moving too close (invading personal space).

In these circumstances, it is difficult not to respond with a primal 'fight or flight' reaction: standing and shouting back, or trying to run from the room. Such extreme reactions are suitable only for the most extreme of situations. In the great majority of cases, the situation can be salvaged and converted to a productive clinical encounter. It can be important to remember that most people do not wish to be angry, nor enjoy feeling out of control, and so they will respond gradually but positively to a calm and controlled response to their outburst. Maintaining a calm demeanour and relaxed posture (at a suitably safe distance, but not backing away), avoiding sudden movements, are essential. A few moments pause before speaking in a calm tone of voice may be sufficient to allow the patient to regain awareness and control of his or her actions. When speaking, focus on the patient's concerns and not on his or her behaviours (for instance, do not insist he or she sits down).

Acknowledging distress

Having recognised the patient's distress, the clinician should acknowledge this as early as possible in the encounter: 'I can see you are very upset (distressed) and I shall do all I can to help you'. An early acknowledgment validates the patient's experience, and goes a long way to overcoming any expectation of rejection, or sensitivity to negative responses, the patient might harbour. In doing so, it might remove the need for unacceptable, over assertive or aggressive expressions. This simple reassurance should not wait until the source of the problem is clear as that may take some time to determine.

Containing distress

Performing in a competent and reliable manner in the face of a patient's distress is a fundamental clinical skill (Box 2.5).

Box 2.5 Practical points in dealing with challenging patients

- Be supportive to patients – explain the options and choices positively
- Apologise when appropriate and necessary
- Take a forgiving attitude to rudeness
- Show you are listening to, and interested in, what the patient says
- Promise only what you have the ability to deliver
- Don't keep agitated patients waiting
- Don't see patients in isolated areas
- Don't become angry when your competence is questioned
- Don't respond in kind (angry, blaming, threatening)
- Don't be patronising or tell patients off
- Don't keep looking at the clock, or the door

The most important element of containment is remaining calm when faced with a patient who is undermining or threatening: 'I'll make a complaint (… get angry, … kill myself)'. These statements are viewed best as a test that the patient (probably on the basis of previous experience) expects the clinician to fail. Failure will ultimately disable the clinician, and reinforce the patient's deep-seated conviction that his or her distress is not amenable to help (or that clinicians are incompetent or dismissive). It helps to remember that pain and distress are felt by the patient, not the clinician.

Containment is reinforced by showing interest in the causes of the patient's distress, and concern for its effects on the patient (and his or her family or acquaintances). This is achieved by gentle probing of the patient's clinical history: 'It will help me if you tell me more about your worries (problems)'. Although the patient may be reluctant (he or she might have been through this process several times in the past), perseverance is important as it maintains the focus on the patient, reinforces the clinician's role, and establishes the basis of their collaboration.

Reflecting distress

An indication of empathy (or sympathetic understanding) shows that although the clinician is not unaffected by the patient's distress, he or she is not overwhelmed by it: 'It must be dreadful for you to feel like this (… to have these feelings)'. Empathic statements assist greatly in containing the patient's distress, and in moving the interview on towards an acceptable conclusion. However, in this as in all aspects of dealing with distressed, angry or difficult patients, it is important to get the balance right. Gushing expressions of concern can easily appear trite or insincere.

A patient's expressions of anger or frustration can be fed back to him or her as questions. 'If I don't get help now, it will be too late', may be rephrased as, 'Are you worried that you might not get the help you need?' Despair that prompts a statement such as, 'You just don't want to help me', may be acknowledged and reflected back by saying, 'Does it seem that doctors never want to help you?' The threat implicit in, 'I'll kill myself and it will be your fault', may be defused to some extent by asking, 'Do you feel that your only option is to kill yourself?'

Modelling appropriate behaviour

People in ordinary conversation will tend to adopt each other's posture and manner: so-called mirroring. However, if a patient expresses his or her distress by standing, pacing, talking loudly or interrupting, a clinician who reacts in kind (or by withdrawing or showing anxiety) may make the patient feel more desperate and so escalate the tension. By remaining calm, attentive and as relaxed as possible, the clinician provides a model for the patient to 'mirror' by adopting a similar demeanour. Not only does this reduce the threat of violence, it facilitates clinical enquiry necessary to deal with the patient's immediate problems.

There are potential longer term benefits. In following these steps, the clinician is modelling appropriate and effective ways of dealing with personal distress. This should mitigate, at least partially, the patient's previous negative experiences of healthcare and encourage future cooperation.

Agreeing achievable goals

All clinical encounters should result in a workable care plan, at very least a simple statement of what will happen next. It is important to summarise the problems from the clinician's perspective, and to agree those that the patient is most concerned to deal with. As patient's and clinician's views might not coincide, it is important to allow some leeway for negotiation. If the interview was too brief to allow a full clinical assessment, then a simple plan is to arrange a longer appointment in the near future to clarify matters.

Once the key issues are agreed, the means of addressing them should be outlined. It will assist if the clinician is aware of what services exist, their referral requirements and waiting lists. Where a patient's problems are long term or recurrent, or require scarce specialist services, wild promises of immediate resolution will be seen as a brush-off and greeted with scorn. A minimum plan will consist of details of what can be offered for each problem, by whom, who will make the arrangements, and in what timescale. It is particularly important to be clear what the clinician will do, and what is expected of the patient. It may help to draw up a short written summary for the patient to take away, as, following a difficult encounter, memories might be unreliable (and a source of future conflict).

Terminating the interview

A final pitfall is ending the interview too abruptly. No matter how busy the clinician, the patient should be given the opportunity to air all outstanding grievances or concerns: if sent away too soon, he or she will feel humiliated and punished, and this will fuel further dissatisfaction. A further appointment – at a definite date and time, not merely 'You may come again' – should be arranged to review progress, to clarify uncertainties (such as progress of any referral), and to check for unresolved issues. Although this may be difficult to arrange if the encounter took place out of normal working hours, it is particularly important as the patient might view continued contact as a demonstration of good faith. For the clinician, it is a statement of his or her competence and confidence in dealing with a challenging situation.

Further information

NHS guidelines on withholding treatment from violent and abusive patients:
- Patients with severe mental health problems or suffering life-threatening conditions will not be denied treatment
- Patients will be offered a verbal warning and a written warning before treatment is withheld: www.nhs.uk/zerotolerance
- Royal College of General Practitioners: 'issues to be considered in the event of apparent irretrievable breakdown of the patient–doctor relationship': www.rcgp.org.uk/corporate/position/removal_of_patients_from_gp_lists1.pdf

Personal account of mental health problems

Haselton A. *Brain injury. A modern medical miracle.* Chipmunkapublishing, Brentwood, Essex, 2006. www.chipmunka.com

Further reading

Houghton A. Handling aggressive patients. *BMJ Careers* 2006; **333**: 63–4. http://careerfocus.bmjjournals.com/cgi/content/full/333/7563/63-a.

Mason T, Chandley M. *Management of violence and aggression: A manual for nurses and health care workers.* Churchill Livingstone, Edinburgh, 1999.

National Institute for Health and Clinical Excellence. *Violence: The short-term management of disturbed/violent behaviour in in-patient psychiatric settings and emergency departments.* NICE guideline CG25. NICE, London, 2005. http://guidance.nice.org.uk/CG25/

NHS Counter Fraud & Security Management Division. *Prevention and management of violence where withdrawal of treatment is not an option.* NHS Business Services Authority, London, 2007. http://www.cfsms.nhs.uk/doc/sms.general/prev_man_violence.pdf

NHS Security Management Service. *Promoting safer and therapeutic services – Implementing the national syllabus in mental health and learning disability services.* NHS SMS, London, 2005. http://www.cfsms.nhs.uk/doc/psts/psts.implementing.syllabus.pdf

Turnbull J, Paterson B (eds). *Managing aggression and violence.* Palgrave Macmillan, Basingstoke, Hampshire, 1999.

Vishwanathan K. Tips on: dealing with angry and aggressive patients. *BMJ Careers* 2006; **333**: 64.

CHAPTER 3

Mental Health Problems in Primary Care

Richard Byng and Jed Boardman

OVERVIEW

- The majority of people with mental health problems are seen in primary care
- Types of problems presenting, and re-presenting, in primary care may differ from the textbook varieties seen by specialists
- General practitioners must detect those features of mental disorder that require treatment, and normalise those that may not benefit from specific mental health interventions
- Current guidelines emphasise the need to contain and treat many mild or moderate mental disorders in primary care, and to collaborate with mental health teams in managing more severe disorders

---

Psychiatric symptoms are common in the general population: worry, tiredness and sleepless nights affect more than half of adults at some time, while as many as one person in seven experiences some form of diagnosable neurotic disorder. The majority of people with mental health problems are seen in primary care (Box 3.1). The preferred method of establishing rates of morbidity is to carry out a systematic survey using a structured or semi-structured interview, possibly combining this with a screening questionnaire in a two-phase process. Two-phase surveys have been carried out in primary care settings in several countries and

---

Box 3.1 **Mental health problems in primary care**

- Emotional symptoms are common but do not necessarily mean that the sufferer has a mental disorder
- Many mood disorders are short lived responses to stresses in people's lives such as bereavement
- About 30% of people with no mental disorder suffer from fatigue, and 12% suffer from depressed mood
- Anxiety and depression often occur together
- Mental disorder comprises about 25% of general practice consultations – in Britain up to 80% of referrals to specialist psychiatric services come from primary care

---

ABC of Mental Health, 2nd edition. Edited by T. Davies and T. Craig.
©2009 Blackwell Publishing, ISBN: 978-0-7279-1639-6.

show variable rates, ranging from 15% to 38.8% depending on the diagnostic criteria used to make the definitive diagnoses. For example, the World Health Organization's study of mental disorder in general healthcare in 14 countries found that a quarter of the 5500 people surveyed had well-defined disorders, the most common of which were depression (10%), generalised anxiety disorder (8%) and harmful use of alcohol (3%).

Psychotic disorders are much less common: approximately 2% of the population have a diagnosis of chronic psychosis, with a sixfold variation between practices; new cases of psychosis (average incidence of less than 1%) present rarely to general practice but are important events requiring early referral to specialist services.

Anxiety and depression, often occurring together, are the most prevalent mental disorders in the general population

---

While population-based studies consistently record high levels of psychiatric disorder, it is not clear to what extent this reflects the met or unmet need for treatment as not everyone who experiences symptoms consults a general practitioner, and of those who do, many do not receive treatment. In the National Survey of Psychiatric Morbidity in Great Britain, only 28.5% of those with neurotic disorders attending primary care were in receipt of treatment. Some people with mental health problems will not want treatment and although stigma for common mental health problems is declining, it is still widespread.

Bereavement

Death of a loved one is a distressing episode in normal human experience. Expression of distress varies greatly between individual people and cultures, but grieving does not constitute mental disorder. The doctor's most appropriate response is compassion and reassurance rather than drug treatment. Night sedation for a few days may be helpful, but over-sedation should be avoided. Antidepressants should be reserved for those patients who develop a depressive episode

Box 3.2 **Main typologies of mental health problems in primary care**

- Acute distress following significant life events (e.g. bereavement)
- Low-grade ongoing mood and anxiety symptoms not meeting criteria for depressive or anxiety disorders, often associated with social adversity
- New episodes of depressive illness or anxiety disorder
- Longstanding chronic or intermittent anxiety and depression often with other psychiatric diagnoses, recurrent self-harm, or substance misuse
- Depression or anxiety associated with long-term physical health problems as the main reason for attending
- Presentation of medically unexplained physical symptoms with possibility of underlying psychological or emotional problems
- New episode of unusual or bizarre behaviour raising possibility of psychosis
- Longstanding psychosis attending with relapse or exacerbation, or with a focus on physical health problems
- Dementia or cognitive decline

Presentation of mental health problems in primary care

Box 3.2 outlines a range of typologies of primary mental healthcare patients; the model is derived by considering medical diagnostic approaches, and incorporating comorbidity and chronicity along with needs for care. The presentation of mental illness to primary care practitioners will be influenced by the patient's understanding of their condition and their previous experience of treatment.

While the role of the general practitioner in detecting the illness has been emphasised, the important role of normalising those who may not benefit from mental health interventions has received far less attention. Primary care practitioners play an important role at the interface between the lay and medical models of mental distress. People presenting with distress lasting days or weeks in response to a significant life event may benefit from reassurance that their symptoms are to be expected. A 'watchful waiting' approach may be all that is required, though always with an eye to problems that fail to resolve or particular patient groups who may be at risk of more severe disorder.

Poor outcome is associated with delayed or insufficient initial treatment, more severe illness, older age at onset, comorbid physical illness, and continuing problems with family, marriage or employment

There is a significant group of patients, many regular attendees in primary care, with chronic anxiety or recurrent depression, making up 5–10% of the consulting population. Likely comorbidities include long-term physical conditions, substance misuse, personality disorders, obsessive–compulsive disorder, post-traumatic stress disorder and eating disorders (Box 3.3). Primary care teams with their ability to provide continuity, reactive care and chronic disease management are in an ideal position to manage this group in collaboration with specialist mental health professionals.

Box 3.3 **Mental disorders presenting with physical complaints**

- Coexisting physical and mental disorders that are essentially independent of each other (such as heart disease in a patient suffering from depression)
- Distress due to physical illness (such as anxiety or depression related to a life-threatening illness)
- Somatic symptoms of a mental disorder (such as palpitations due to anxiety)
- Chronic somatisation disorders in which patients express hypochondriacal convictions that physical disease is present in the absence of any medical evidence for this

Box 3.4 **Important components of consultations for mental health problems**

- Listen to narrative
- Engage in a conversation encompassing psychological or emotional distress
- Elicit ideas and beliefs about well-being and mental illness
- Reach a mutually agreed formulation or diagnosis in medical and/or social terms
- Make a risk assessment
- Be positive while acknowledging difficulties
- Provide information about a range of management options – medication, talking therapy, and social or health promoting strategies
- Elicit concerns and expectations about treatments
- Reach a shared decision about a management plan
- Reinforce the contribution of the patient to his or her own care (self-care)
- Arrange review and follow-up
- Look after your own emotions

Recognition and engagement

Box 3.4 illustrates a framework, influenced by models of GP consultations, for managing mental health problems in primary care. Problems may be recognised by both the GP and the patient, but not necessarily simultaneously. Achieving recognition by a mutual agreement about diagnosis and understanding about the patient's emotional distress appears to involve a number of important stages. Talk about emotional issues may be embedded within consultations about physical health. Both patient and practitioner may dance around the possibility of entering an in-depth discussion about the emotional elements, perhaps due to stigma or perhaps for fear of upsetting an existing comfortable relationship. Continuity may help, or sometimes hinder, the process of engagement with the emotional, and with making a diagnosis of mental illness.

Listening to narrative and subtly encouraging talk about psychosocial issues may also be an important prerequisite to achieving mutual acknowledgment about emotional distress (emotional expression in therapy has been linked to remission). Once achieved, the conversation will need to address the patient's ideas and beliefs about the cause of his or her own distress, and whether he or she sees the problem as being part of 'the cares of life' – a social model, biochemical phenomena or genetic predisposition. This understanding will help a practitioner to gain trust and explain mental illness and its treatment in terms accepted and understood by the patient.

Medical practitioners do have an important role in making a diagnosis, but it does not always need to be pivotal. A diagnosis can be helpful for some patients: as a way of feeling understood; to feel less isolated; to explain their symptoms and distress; or to obtain sick notes. In some conditions it helps define the optimal treatment. There may be differences of opinion, with the practitioner wishing to normalise or demedicalise a condition and a patient wanting something done perhaps in the form of a prescription for medication. Alternatively, the patient may be reluctant to enter into the medical realm and accept a psychiatric diagnosis. Being open about these differences of opinion is part of a concordant consultation.

Risk assessment is required to ensure that significant risk of self-harm or suicide are managed (Box 3.5). It is also worth considering the possibility of harm to others, and in primary care this is most likely related to the patient's ability to care for dependents, particularly children. Other chapters in this book will provide detailed accounts of how specific conditions can be diagnosed accurately, whereas this framework has focused on how, in the context of primary care, comorbidity and past history affect the process of engagement with the psychosocial elements of distress.

Managing mental disorder

Guidance from the National Institute for Health and Clinical Excellence (NICE) places increasing emphasis on management of mental health problems in primary care. Management options for mental health problems can be divided broadly into health promoting activities, psychological therapies and medication. All of these involve elements of self-care and sharing responsibility with the patient. The 'stepped care' model for depression and anxiety provides a framework for rationing intensity (and cost) of treatment against need. The NICE guidance for depression has usefully uncoupled the diagnosis from the imperative to provide medication with the insertion of a period of 'watchful waiting' (Box 3.6). The term is a misnomer, however, and rarely involves doing nothing. In fact, this period might include the use of basic counselling approaches, normalisation of distress in response to life events, reattribution of somatic symptoms for those with medically unexplained symptoms, and the provision of health promoting advice about exercise, substance misuse, sleep and sensible work patterns. These may require skilful psychological manoeuvres by generalist clinicians embedded within short consultations.

For those being considered for more complex and costly treatment, an explanation about the proposed treatment (possibly with the help of written information sheets or internet websites) combined with a dialogue about the patient's concerns and expectations about treatment is an essential foundation for shared decision-making. More patients are likely to receive effective treatments if choice of treatment modality is based on their beliefs, expectations and convenience, rather than treatments being prescribed purely on the basis of the currently insufficient evidence matching treatment to specific conditions. The stepped care approach to the organisation of psychosocial interventions allows a number of options for each level of need in order, for example, to save longer term and specialist therapies for those not responding to antidepressants and briefer treatment.

Specialist input is one of the pillars of chronic disease management, and referral to secondary care has been seen as an important function of the primary care consultation (Box 3.7). Onward referral to outpatient psychiatry clinics has largely been replaced by an array of mechanisms for achieving specialist support that includes: referral for assessment by community mental health teams; email or telephone consultation; consultation liaison; primary care-based counsellors and therapists; practice-based community mental health nurses (formerly community psychiatric nurses, CPNs), occupational therapists and social workers. Despite evidence for efficacy of psychological interventions in common mental disorders, there is a significant shortage of therapists, particularly in primary care.

Safety netting and reviewing care

Proactive review of care has been shown to improve outcomes for people with mental health problems. Safety netting at the end of a consultation and ensuring that care is reviewed is relevant to the range of presentations within primary care, and is established as a key component of the consultation. For those thought likely to have self-limiting conditions, a critical component of normalisation, or referral to care away from specialist care settings, is to ensure that if problems worsen the patient feels empowered to return for review. For those with common mental health problems, such as single episodes of depression, there is increasing, although not conclusive, evidence that follow-up in primary care should be more proactive, using procedures such as medication adherence education and telephone reviews.

Patients with complex long-term mental health problems, even if in contact with specialist mental health services, will still benefit from a primary care-based review. This should be integrated with systems of chronic disease management for physical health problems, such as diabetes and cardiovascular disease, that are at increased risk as comorbid conditions with severe mental illness. Many older patients with dementia and chronic depression will also fall into this category. This proactive care would incorporate a range of options, including an emphasis on self-care, timely support from specialist mental health workers, signposting to community resources, referral for brief episodes of therapy, involvement of carers and family, and the development of crisis and recovery plans.

Supporting the development of primary care mental health systems

Advances in information technology may increase access to knowledge about mental health and its treatment for both patients and professionals. This will provide increasingly a range of treatment options for some groups, and will support systems for reviewing care, with web-based recall systems and databases about individual patients. While supervision has been accepted as a requirement for specialist mental health workers, generalist primary care workers, such as GPs and nurses, have often lacked the support required to ensure high-quality care is maintained. Finally, it may be important to support the practitioners suffering 'burnout' or poor personal mental health in order to ensure that patients registered with their practices receive adequate primary care-based mental healthcare.

Further reading

Bebbington P, Brugha TS, Meltzer H, *et al.* Neurotic disorders and the receipt of psychiatric treatment. *Psychol Med* 2000; **30:** 1369–76.

Bebbington P, Meltzer H, Brugha TS, *et al.* Unequal access and unmet need: neurotic disorders and the use of primary care services. *Psychol Med* 2000; **30:** 1359–67.

Boardman J, Parsonage M. *Delivering the government's mental health policies. Services, staffing and costs.* Sainsbury Centre for Mental Health, London, 2007.

Boardman J, Willmott S, Henshaw C. The prevalence of the needs for mental health treatment in general practice attenders. *Br J Psych* 2004; **185:** 318–27.

Goldberg D, Huxley P. *Mental illness in the community. The pathway to psychiatric care.* Tavistock, London, 1980.

National Institute for Health and Clinical Excellence. *Anxiety (amended): Management of anxiety (panic disorder, with or without agoraphobia, and generalised anxiety disorder) in adults in primary, secondary and community care.* NICE guideline CG22. NICE, London, 2007. http://guidance.nice.org.uk/CG22/

National Institute for Health and Clinical Excellence. *Depression (amended): Management of depression in primary and secondary care.* NICE guideline CG23. NICE, London, 2007. http://guidance.nice.org.uk/CG23/

Ustun TB, Sartorius N (eds). *Mental illness in general health care.* Wiley, Chichester, 1995.

CHAPTER 4

Managing Mental Health Problems in the General Hospital

Amanda Ramirez and Allan House

> **OVERVIEW**
>
> - Mental health problems of general hospital patients are closely tied to their physical illness, and especially prevalent in some specialties
> - Patients who self-harm may require brief admission, and medical management should be followed by a psychosocial assessment by specially trained staff
> - Acute psychiatric disorders may occur in any patient with a physical illness, and those with severe, painful or disfiguring illnesses (or treatments) are at greatest risk
> - Suspect psychiatric problems in those who have medically unexplained symptoms, fail to adhere to treatment, or develop unexpected disability

The prevalence of mental health problems in patients attending acute general hospitals is high (Box 4.1). The three main types of clinical problem are

- Acute presentations of psychiatric disorder, including self-harm and other psychiatric crises and emergencies
- Psychiatric disorder in patients with physical illness
- Psychologically based physical syndromes (somatisation).

All doctors have a role in addressing the mental health needs of their patients. Mental health problems of general hospital patients are closely tied to their physical illness, and specialist units (such as cancer, renal, pain, neurology or AIDS services) may experience a high level of psychiatric disorder. Patients, and staff, benefit from specific psychiatric liaison support to facilitate integration of their psychological and physical care.

Acute presentations of psychiatric disorder

Self-harm

About 150,000 cases of self-harm present to accident and emergency departments annually in the United Kingdom. Most of these acts of self-harm involve self-poisoning, and nearly half of these involve paracetamol overdose. About 20% of patients injure

> Box 4.1 **Prevalence of mental health problems in general hospitals**
>
> - Hospital attendances for self-harm average 150–200 per 100,000 population. A district general hospital with a population of 250,000 will have about 500 attendees a year. In central London 11% of acute adult medical admissions follow deliberate self-harm
> - Up to 5% of patients attending emergency departments have psychiatric symptoms alone, but 20–30% have important psychiatric symptoms coexisting with physical disorder
> - Patients with serious physical illness have at least twice the rate of psychiatric disorder found in the general population: 20–40% of all hospital outpatients and inpatients have an important psychiatric disorder
> - A quarter of new outpatients to a medical clinic have no important relevant physical disease: 9–12% of referrals of medical outpatients may involve somatisation

themselves in other ways, usually by cutting. Alcohol consumption forms a part of about 45% of episodes of self-harm.

Among patients attending hospital with self-harm, men and women are nearly equally represented and the average age is about 30 years. For most, the act is a response to social and interpersonal problems such as housing or work-related problems, unemployment, debt and conflicts in relationships. Only a minority have severe mental illness.

About 20% of patients attend hospital again within a year of harming themselves and 0.5–1% commit suicide. In England and Wales, about 1000 people a year commit suicide within 12 months of a general hospital attendance for non-fatal self-harm – almost a quarter of the total annual suicides. The national targets for reducing suicide could be met entirely by halving the suicide rate after hospital attendance for self-harm.

Managing self-harm

Integrated management of such patients is facilitated by overnight admission to a short-stay ward, even when this is not medically indicated. This provides the opportunity for adequate psychosocial assessment, including family involvement in the process, and temporary respite from the precipitating crisis. Some patients may, of course, decline admission but should be assessed as fully as possible before they leave hospital (Box 4.2).

ABC of Mental Health, 2nd edition. Edited by T. Davies and T. Craig. © 2009 Blackwell Publishing, ISBN: 978-0-7279-1639-6.

Assessing self-harm

All patients presenting with self-harm benefit from a psychosocial assessment by staff specifically trained for this task. This and other aspects of the care of people who present to hospital after self-harm have been the subject of recent NICE guidelines on good practice (Box 4.3). The assessment has two functions. Firstly, the sizeable minority of patients who have a psychiatric disorder (usually mood disorder or clinically important substance misuse) can be identified. These patients benefit from standard psychiatric treatment.

Secondly, it provides an opportunity to understand a patient's predicament in a way that integrates symptoms and mental state with information about social and interpersonal difficulties. Full assessment of the context in which an individual episode has occurred improves accurate diagnosis and reduces the inappropriate and pejorative use of diagnostic terms such as 'personality disorder'.

Intervention after self-harm is intended to improve the social adjustment and personal well-being of patients and may reduce the risk of repetition. Brief individual therapy based on a problem-solving approach is of most value (Box 4.4). For people who present repeatedly after self-harm, two approaches have been suggested: a specialist form of psychotherapy known as dialectical behaviour therapy (DBT), and a structured approach to harm minimisation for those whose presentations involve self-cutting.

Box 4.2 **Risk groups for self-harm**

Patients at high risk
- Those with psychiatric disorder, including: major affective disorder, substance misuse, schizophrenia
- But they constitute only a small proportion of cases

Patients at lower risk
- Those with social and personal problems who are poor problem solvers due to lack of support, previous abuse or neglect
- They constitute a large proportion of cases

Box 4.3 **Features of a service to manage self-harm**

- Brief admission available to all as an option
- Early psychosocial assessment by specially trained and supervised staff after initial medical management
- Immediate access to psychiatric care where appropriate
- Early follow-up by multidisciplinary team, with outreach or domiciliary visits when necessary
- Good communication and liaison with medical and surgical teams, general practitioners and other agencies

---

Box 4.4 **Therapy based on problem solving**

This includes teaching patients to
- Identify problems and arrange priorities for problem solving
- Generate a wide range of solutions
- Narrow this down to concrete and attainable goals that would represent a personally important improvement
- Work out and implement steps to achieving goals, together with ways of determining and maintaining success

---

Box 4.5 **Types of acute psychiatric problem that may present in hospitals**

- Acute psychiatric disturbance (such as paranoid states, mania, delirium, panic)
- Alcohol and drug misuse, including delirium tremens
- Problems of adjustment to chronic physical illness leading to repeated hospital attendance (such as for asthma, diabetes or epilepsy)
- Mood disorder (such as anxiety states, depression)
- Personal crises

Other psychiatric crises and emergencies

Emergency departments of acute general hospitals are commonly the first port of call for people in crisis. The use of an emergency department by psychiatric patients depends on the organisation of acute general psychiatry services. The proportion of attendees with psychiatric problems is greatly increased if the emergency department is a 'place of safety' to which the police may bring a person who seems to be suffering from mental disorder under the Mental Health Act. Many types of acute psychiatric problem may present to an accident and emergency department or occur among inpatients on the wards (Box 4.5).

Managing psychiatric crises and emergencies

Assessment of these patients is similar to the approach outlined for patients with self-harm. This can be undertaken effectively by a psychiatric nurse, who coordinates subsequent care with the relevant agencies, including the liaison psychiatrist, general psychiatric services and social services. Policies about length of stay in emergency departments – such as the '4-hour rule' – impose organisational (rather than clinical) challenges, and negotiation is required between emergency department staff, the liaison team and local crisis resolution services to ensure that a rapid and effective response is made.

Psychiatric disorder associated with physical illness

Psychiatric disorder may be a consequence of physical illness (such as mood disorder in cancer patients), a cause (such as alcohol misuse leading to pancreatitis), or a coincidental occurrence. Less than half of the psychiatric disorder in physically ill patients is recognized and treated appropriately (Box 4.6).

- Mood disorder – mainly anxiety and depression in association with life-threatening illness, chronic disability or hospitalisation. Two-thirds of mood disorders resolve as part of the normal process of adjustment to physical illness. A third do not improve unless specifically addressed and so require active treatment
- Alcohol- and drug-related problems – alcohol contributes indirectly to many conditions that present to acute general hospitals, particularly gastrointestinal, liver and neurological disorders. Drug-related problems include hepatitis, infective endocarditis and HIV infection
- Organic brain disease – mental disorder may be associated with brain disease (such as stroke, head injury and epilepsy).

Box 4.6 **Identifying psychiatric disorder in physically ill patients**

Physical illness with high risk of psychiatric disorder
- Severe, life-threatening disease
- Painful, stressful or disfiguring treatment
Unexplained poor outcome of physical illness
- Poor adherence to treatment
- Excessive handicap
- Multiple symptoms or presentations
Patients with high risk of psychiatric disorder
- Previous psychiatric history
- Poor social support
Concurrent psychological symptoms
- Worries
- Anxiety symptoms
- Depressive symptoms

Box 4.7 **Psychological problems that may be associated with physical illness**

- Poor adherence to advice or treatment (such as for diabetes, asthma, sickle cell disease)
- Unexplained handicap, when functional disability after an acute illness is out of proportion to physical impairment
- Sexual dysfunction, which may result from a complex interplay of several factors (emotional impact of the illness, general debility, metabolic and hormonal changes, autonomic and arterial disease, and side effects of prescribed drugs)
- Body image disorders after mutilating surgery (such as colostomy, limb amputation, mastectomy, surgery for head and neck cancer)
- Eating disorders, including anorexia and bulimia nervosa, and obesity (such as in diabetics)

Box 4.8 **Basic psychological skills for all clinicians**

All hospital clinicians should be able to
- Communicate clearly with patients, discuss concerns and elicit misapprehensions and correct them
- Break bad news in a honest, compassionate and timely way
- Facilitate grieving by patients and their relatives
- Discuss psychological symptoms and distress without embarrassment
- Discuss the need for specialist psychiatric help without seeming dismissive
- Use antidepressants rationally

Box 4.9 **Treatments for psychiatric disorder in physically ill patients**

- Brief psychological treatments delivered by trained staff are effective and include grief work, cognitive behavioural therapy, behaviour therapy and interpersonal psychotherapy
- Non-specific 'counselling' and 'support' are of limited benefit in managing clinically important psychological problems
- Antidepressant drugs are beneficial in patients with conspicuous mood disorder. Tricyclic antidepressants and selective serotonin reuptake inhibitors have similar efficacy but different toxicity profiles. Choice of drug should take account of patients' physical symptoms (for example, tricyclics may benefit those with pain and insomnia but should be avoided in patients with prostatism)

Missing from this list is the provision of self-help materials and advice, as, although their provision would be desirable, there is little available for most people – computer and web-based resources being accessible only by a minority.

Treating psychiatric disorder in physically ill patients

The cornerstone of treatment is psychological therapy, either alone or in conjunction with psychotropic drugs (Box 4.9). There are a number of candidate therapies: individual (cognitive behavioural therapy (CBT), interpersonal), family or group-based. In practice, the available treatments are not exclusive and can be modified according to the needs of each patient. For example, in some patients undergoing CBT, an intrusive marital problem may emerge that requires the introduction of marital or family therapy. Psychiatrists must be alert to the development or progression of organic disease and collaborate with the medical team in developing a management strategy.

Psychologically based physical syndromes (somatisation)

Many patients referred to hospital for investigation of physical symptoms do not have an identifiable physical disorder that explains their symptoms. About a quarter of new cases of abdominal pain in gastroenterology clinics and atypical chest pain in cardiology clinics, and most general practice referrals to neurology, have no relevant physical disease. Many of these patients do not respond to

Other psychological problems that may be associated with physical illness include poor adherence to advice or treatment, unexplained handicap, sexual dysfunction, body image disorders and eating disorders (Box 4.7).

Management strategies for all patients with physical illness

All clinicians can act to minimise psychological distress in their patients. A useful model is the stepped care approach recommended for the management of depression in primary care. Underpinning this approach is good face-to-face communication between clinicians and patients and carers, for which effective communication skills training is a prerequisite (Box 4.8).

Components include:
- Identifying worries and concerns (whether accurate or inaccurate)
- Providing factual information and educating patients about their illness and its management
- Encouraging appropriate expression of anxiety and distress
- Involvement of family and close others in discussions about the illness and its impact, when at all possible
- Reviewing patients to identify any persistent worries and mood symptoms, using a simple self-report questionnaire if desired
- Referring patients with persistent psychological difficulties to mental health services.

> **Box 4.10 Management strategies for patients with unexplained physical symptoms**
>
> It is important that
> - Patients' symptoms and their understanding of these symptoms are elicited in full
> - Psychosocial cues are identified and explored (such as low mood, distressing events and personal difficulties)
> - Symptoms and investigations are reviewed – telling patients that 'nothing is wrong' is not helpful, but negative findings and their implications should be discussed (for example, 'There is no evidence that your symptoms are due to cancer')
> - Clinicians then explain to patients that their physical symptoms may have a psychological origin (for example, tension headaches, hyperventilation and tachycardia may all be manifestations of anxiety). This can be linked to current psychosocial problems that have been elicited
> - Management plans can then be reviewed with patients, and limits set on further investigations and drug prescribing
> - Revised plans are communicated to the patient's general practitioner to avoid misunderstandings and 'doctor shopping'
> - Referral to mental health services is considered

reassurance and, if discharged, are referred to another department or another hospital. Most of these patients have psychological factors underlying their illness.

Somatisation

The presentation of psychosocial distress as physical complaints has costs to the patients, their relatives and the health service, particularly in severe and chronic cases. It is associated with a burden of physical and psychosocial disabilities for patients and their relatives. It is costly in terms of unnecessary investigation and treatment, loss of income, iatrogenic problems and unnecessary welfare benefits.

All clinicians should be able to undertake the initial management of such cases: introducing early in care the idea that in many cases investigation does not yield a biomedical explanation for illnesses; communicating clearly to prevent repeated and excessive investigation.

Psychological treatment of unexplained physical symptoms

There are several psychological approaches to treating unexplained physical symptoms; the better evaluated are based on the principles of CBT.

Clinical characteristics may have a bearing on the particular type of psychological treatment used. For example, markedly abnormal behaviour (such as staying in bed all day) indicates that behavioural treatment might be appropriate (such as graded activity). Cognitive treatment might be better suited to patients with dysfunctional beliefs such as, 'Investigations should be able to find the cause of my symptoms', or, 'It is unsafe to do anything on my own'.

For patients who do not respond or refuse psychological help, an approach to containment of demands for investigation and treatment may need to be negotiated, which must include the general practitioner (Box 4.10).

Personal accounts of mental health problems

Haselton A. *A modern medical miracle*. Chipmunkapublishing, Brentwood, Essex, 2006. www.chipmunka.com

Pymer L. *Emotional thump*. Chipmunkapublishing, Brentwood, Essex, 2007. www.chipmunka.com

Rainbow J. *Don't cut my life-line*. Chipmunkapublishing, Brentwood, Essex, 2006. www.chipmunka.com

Further reading

Creed F, Mayou R, Hopkins A (eds). *Medical symptoms not explained by organic disease*. Royal College of Psychiatrists, Royal College of Physicians of London, London, 1992.

Fallowfield L, Jenkins V, Farewell V, *et al*. Efficacy of a Cancer Research UK communication skills training model for oncologists: a randomized controlled trial. *Lancet* 2002; **359**: 650–6.

Gask L, Morriss R. Assessment and immediate management of people at risk of harming themselves. *Psychiatry* 2006; **5**: 266–70.

National Institute for Health and Clinical Excellence. *Guidance on cancer services. Improving supportive and palliative care for adults with cancer. The manual*. NICE, London, 2004. http://www.nice.org.uk/nicemedia/pdf/csg-spmanual.pdf

National Institute for Health and Clinical Excellence. *Self-harm: The short-term physical and psychological management and secondary prevention of self-harm in primary and secondary care*. NICE guideline CG16. NICE, London, 2004. http://guidance.nice.org.uk/CG16/

National Institute for Health and Clinical Excellence. *Management of depression in primary and secondary care*. NICE guideline CG23. NICE, London, 2004. http://guidance.nice.org.uk/CG23/

National Institute for Health and Clinical Excellence. *Management of chronic fatigue /myalgic encephalitis*. NICE guideline CG53. NICE, London, 2007. http://guidance.nice.org.uk/CG53/

CHAPTER 5

Mental Health Emergencies

Zerrin Atakan and David Taylor

OVERVIEW

- Mental health emergencies occur in all clinical and community settings, so preparation and prediction are key components of management
- The first consideration in dealing with emergencies, whether violent or not, is the safety of all concerned
- Essential emergency treatments are sanctioned by the common law, but ongoing assessment and treatment may require detention under the Mental Health Act
- Guidelines exist for rapid tranquillisation under medical supervision to control potentially destructive behaviour, when non-pharmacological methods have failed

---

A mental health emergency is a situation that requires immediate attention to avert a serious outcome, which may arise from a range of situations where a patient is at risk because of intense personal distress, suicidal intentions, or self-neglect to those where a patient places others at risk. Some patients may behave in an aggressive manner, make threats or act violently. Such behaviour may produce physical or psychological injury in other people or damage property (Box 5.1).

Causes of mental health emergencies

What makes a situation an emergency depends on the individual patient and the circumstances. Contrary to the general impression, patients with mental disorders are more often the victims than the perpetrators of violence. They are often feared by the public, and this may render them vulnerable to assault. A patient's own health is often at risk from his or her behaviour, as in attempted suicide or severe depression. Other people may be more at risk of neglect or accidental involvement than of intentional violence.

In difficult circumstances almost any patient may behave violently and pose a risk to their own safety or that of others. Not all emergencies involve psychotic disorders. Neurotic disorders such as acute anxiety or panic disorder can cause chaotic or dangerous behaviour. Substance or alcohol use may increase disinhibition especially for risk-taking behaviour and propensity to violence.

ABC of Mental Health, 2nd edition. Edited by T. Davies and T. Craig.
© 2009 Blackwell Publishing, ISBN: 978-0-7279-1639-6.

Box 5.1 **Examples of mental health emergencies**

Immediate risk to a patient's health and well being
- Nihilistic delusions or depressive stupor (stops eating and drinking)
- Manic excitement (stops eating, becomes exhausted and dehydrated)
- Self-neglect (depression, dementia)
- Vulnerability to assault or exploitation (substance misuse and many mental disorders)
- Sexual exploitation

Immediate risk to a patient's safety
- Suicidal intentions (plans and preparations, especially if concealed from others)
- Deliberate self-harm (as result of personality disorder, delusional beliefs or poor coping skills)
- Chaotic behaviour (during intense anxiety, panic, psychosis)

Immediate risk to others
- To family (due to depressive or paranoid delusions)
- To children, who may be neglected due to parent's erratic behaviour (in schizophrenia or mania)
- To newborn baby (in postnatal depression or puerperal psychosis)
- To general public (due to paranoid or persecutory delusions or passivity symptoms such as delusions of being controlled by a specific person)

Safety and risk

Preventing violent incidents has two main components: preparation and prediction.

Preparation

This requires constant awareness of potential risks and hazards to personal safety and of the need to maintain a safe environment. The design and layout of the clinic or surgery should be as pleasant and relaxing as possible – patients do react according to their environment. Dead ends, blind spots and potential weapons should be minimised. All staff should receive regular training in personal safety and emergency procedures.

Dealing with emergencies in the community can be particularly difficult. Just as for medical emergencies, the ability of the lone general practitioner to manage a situation may be limited: the priority is to raise the alarm and obtain assistance without delay (Box 5.2).

Patients may feel threatened and frightened in the alien environment of the inpatient setting. Patients and their carers should be listened to and time spent creating a trusting relationship in which the patient starts to feel safe and cared for. This is crucial, as most violent incidents occurring on inpatient units are due to poor communication and not meeting these basic needs.

Prediction and prevention of violence

This requires awareness of the risks posed by a specific patient or situation (Box 5.3). It is always best to predict accurately, as far as possible, and prevent an incident before it starts or escalates.

Short-term prediction

It is usually easier to predict an incident in the short term when a patient is highly aroused and threatening. Worsening of symptoms, especially delusions or hallucinations that focus on a particular person, can be predictive. Other warning signs will vary from patient to patient and may not be reliable. These include changes or extremes of behaviour (shouting or whispering), outward signs of inner tension (clenched fists, pacing, slamming doors) and repetition of previous behaviour patterns associated with violence. Prior knowledge and avoidance of specific circumstances or conditions that may make a particular individual violent can also be very useful in preventing an incident.

Long-term prediction

Although its reliability is poor, the best long-term predictor of a person's propensity for violence is a history of violent behaviour. Knowledge of a patient's patterns of behaviour, and of what triggers violence, are of greatest importance. This requires careful recording of incidents and clear communication between staff and other agencies. Risk-assessment tools should be used and updated regularly.

The violent incident

The first consideration in dealing with emergencies, whether violent or not, is the safety of all concerned. Actions taken in good faith to avert imminent disaster are sanctioned by common law and do not require recourse to the Mental Health Act. Formal detention and admission to hospital for continued treatment may be considered later.

Rapid tranquillisation

Rapid tranquillisation (RT) is the short-term use of tranquillising drugs to control potentially destructive behaviour. It should be used only under medical supervision and when other, non-pharmacological, methods have failed. Most patients can be 'talked down' and distracted and attempts must be made first to achieve the calming down of the patient. Staff should be trained in using de-escalation techniques to prevent the use of rapid tranquillisation, which may be a traumatic event for the patient, his carers and the staff who are applying it. However, there may be situations when rapid tranquillisation must be considered immediately when safety for all is in danger. In most patients, the precipitating symptoms of arousal (tension and anxiety, excitement and hyperactivity) respond to adequate drug treatment in a few hours.

As far as possible, an assessment of the patient's background, and psychiatric, medical and drug history should be available and a physical examination should have been carried out. Drug allergies and significant medical problems should be checked. Concurrent oral and depot medication should be noted to avoid overdosing and polypharmacy.

In most situations patients accept oral medication and this should be offered first. Where this is not successful, intramuscular administration should be considered. Before administering drugs, ensure that the patient is securely restrained. Staff must be properly trained in using safe methods of restraint. Injecting a struggling patient risks inadvertent intravasation or intra-arterial injection (causing necrosis), damage to sciatic nerve (if the buttock is the chosen site) or other injury.

- Time – Do not rush, allow time for the patient to calm down. Most patients can be 'talked down' in time. Engaging patients in conversation and allowing them to vent their grievances may be all that is required
- Manner – Talk calmly. Reassure patients that you will help them to control themselves, as aroused patients can be frightened of their own destructive potential. Try to find the cause of the present situation, but avoid heated confrontation. Explain your intentions to the patient and all others present. Be clear, direct, non-threatening and honest as this will help confused and aroused patients to calm themselves
- Posture – Stand sideways on to the patient: this is less threatening and presents a smaller target. Keep your hands visible so that it is obvious you are not concealing a weapon
- Staff – Trying to cope alone can lead to disaster. Adequate numbers of staff, preferably trained in dealing with such situations, should be available to restrain the patient and contain the incident. In the community, this means summoning help before attempting to deal with a violent situation.

Medication used in rapid tranquillisation

There is no strong evidence base for medication used in rapid tranquillisation, largely because patients are too disturbed to consent to research. Therefore, the recommendations are based partly on research data, partly on theoretical considerations, but also on clinical experience (Box 5.4).

Recently, there have been two large, randomised controlled trials by the TREC Collaborative Group, which have investigated the efficacy of some intramuscular rapid tranquillisation medications in acutely disturbed patients. All treatment options were effective; however, TREC 1 found midazolam 7.5–15 mg to be more rapidly sedating than a combination of haloperidol 5 or 10 mg and promethazine 50 mg. TREC 2 found haloperidol 10 mg combined with promethazine 25 or 50 mg to be more rapidly sedating than lorazepam 4 mg. Adverse effects were uncommon with all regimens despite the use of somewhat higher doses than might be seen in routine clinical practice.

A flow chart to guide the use of medication in RT is given in Figure 5.1.

After the incident: aftercare

After intramuscular or intravenous administration of drugs, patients should continue to be restrained until they show signs of calming down: further doses might be required. Patients who accept oral tranquillisation should be allowed to calm down in a quiet room. When sedated, patients should be placed in the recovery position and their heart rate, respiration and blood pressure should be monitored regularly. Pulse oximetry is advised for patients who

---

Box 5.4 **Some rapid tranquillisation medications**

- Haloperidol: 5–10 mg IM initially, repeated if required after 30–60 minutes. IV use not recommended: sudden death and cardiac arrest reported
- Zuclopenthixol acetate: not licensed nor suitable for RT. Usual dose is 50–150 mg IM with onset of action in 3 hours and attainment of peak effects over several more hours. Maximum four injections and 400 mg per 'course' (a rather unhelpful concept in RT). Cardiotoxic and high risk especially when given to a highly aroused, struggling patient. Sudden death has been reported. Not found to be superior to haloperidol or other RT medications. However, may be preferred when multiple injections need to be avoided
- Olanzapine: 5–10 mg IM, repeated if required after 30 or 60 minutes. Studies that compare its efficacy against haloperidol suggest that it is faster acting
- Benzodiazepines: not licensed for RT. As well as providing sedation, enhance dopamine-mediated transmission and possibly provide an antipsychotic effect. Respiratory depression is a risk and flumazenil should be readily available. Lorazepam, diazepam and midazolam are the benzodiazepines most commonly used in RT
  - Lorazepam 1–2 mg IM is commonly used in combination with haloperidol
  - Diazepam 10 mg IV is used when very rapid response is required. Diazepam is not used IM
  - Midazolam 7.5–15 mg is a suitable alternative to lorazepam
- Available evidence suggests a combination of a benzodiazepine and an antipsychotic gives superior efficacy to either medication used alone

Other drugs:
- Amylobarbitone IM may sometimes be used in specialist units after consulting a senior clinician
- Paraldehyde is sometimes used in exceptional circumstances

---

lose consciousness. All should be observed continuously until ambulatory.

Everyone involved in a violent or distressing incident, including the patient and any onlookers, may suffer psychological distress. For example, the victim of an assault may go through several phases, being initially numbed or 'shocked', later showing anger or emotional distress, and finally succumbing to mental and physical exhaustion. Others may show some of these reactions. Ample time should be allowed for all involved to talk about the incident and the reasons why rapid tranquillisation was required.

- Treating injuries – Any physical injuries sustained during the incident by the patient, staff or others should be examined and treated
- Recording the incident – The details of the incident should be carefully recorded and reported to the appropriate authority. All services, including primary care and community teams, should have specific procedures for this. Staff involved in the incident may require help in recording their involvement. Staff may be reluctant to report minor injuries or damage to the police, but their rights to compensation may be compromised if they do not
- Involving the police – The police should always be informed if a criminal offence has been committed or weapons have been used.

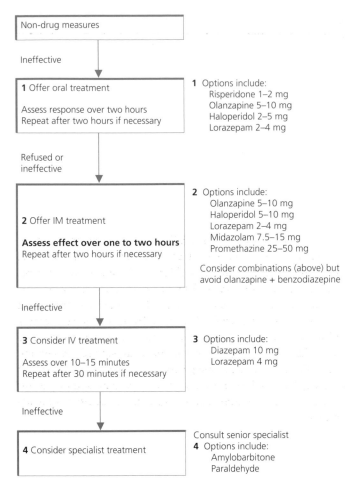

Figure 5.1 Flow chart for rapid control of the acutely disturbed patient (rapid tranquillisation). This chart is for guidance only, rigid adherence to it may not always be appropriate.

It is usually in the interests of the public and patients to deal with offending behaviour through the legal system

• Debriefing – All staff involved should assemble a day or two later to discuss the incident, support each other and glean any lessons that may be learned.

Suicidal patients

Usually, suicidal patients will talk about their intentions: they should be interviewed sensitively but fully about the frequency and intensity of suicidal ideas and about preparations and immediate plans. Their intentions should be viewed in the context of their current circumstances (precipitating events, losses, social support), history (previous self-harm or suicide attempts, known mental or personality disorder) and mental state (depressed, angry, deluded, pessimistic). Those who show clear suicidal intent may need admission to hospital: they should be supervised until their suicidal ideation diminishes in intensity and be given the opportunity to talk of their anguish.

Patients intent on suicide may present a danger to others as well as themselves. They may need to be restrained physically or tranquillised, and all the considerations of safety and follow-up mentioned above apply. Profoundly depressed patients, even if showing severe motor and cognitive slowing (retardation), may react with unexpected physical arousal at attempts to intervene.

Major incidents

After a major incident, such as a train crash or a bombing, it is now customary to provide counselling for all those involved. Evidence suggests that this may not be necessary for everyone, and may be detrimental to some, but deciding who requires such a form of support is difficult in the face of an overwhelming tragedy. Psychological and specialist psychiatric help should be available to those deemed by the emergency services to need it. This will include members of the emergency services themselves. Post-traumatic stress disorder may not be evident for weeks or even months after a serious incident.

Further reading

Alexander J *et al*. Rapid tranquillization of violent or agitated patients in a psychiatric emergency setting. Pragmatic randomised trial of intramuscular lorazepam v. haloperidol plus promethazine. *Br J Psych* 2004; **185**: 63–9.

Battaglia J. Pharmacological management of acute agitation. *Drugs* 2005; **65**: 1207–22.

Holmes, CL, Simmons H, Pilowsky LS. Rapid tranquillisation. In: Beer DM, Pereira SM, Paton C, eds. *Psychiatric intensive care*. Greenwich Medical Books, London, 2001: 42–58.

Huf G, Coutinho ES, Adams CE. TREC-Rio trial: a randomised controlled trial for rapid tranquillisation for agitated patients in emergency psychiatric rooms. *BMC Psych* 2002; **2**: 11.

Taylor D, Paton C, Kerwin R. Acutely disturbed or violent behaviour. In: Taylor D, Paton C, Kerwin R, eds. *The Maudsley prescribing guidelines*, 8th edn. Taylor & Francis, London, 2005: 313–15.

TREC Collaborative Group. Rapid tranquillisation for agitated patients in emergency psychiatric rooms: a randomised trial of midazolam versus haloperidol plus promethazine. *BMJ* 2003; **327**: 708–13.

CHAPTER 6

Mental Health Services

Rosalind Ramsay and Frank Holloway

OVERVIEW

- The UK provides less mental healthcare in specialist settings than most comparable countries

- Most secondary mental healthcare is provided by generic community mental health teams, complemented by a range of specialist 'functional' teams

- Community mental health teams bridge the divide between varied sources of referrals and the complexity of secondary mental health services

- Movement between primary and secondary care relies on thresholds of need: particular diagnoses, complex needs, comorbidity and risk

- Care Programme Approach provides a framework for care of patients accepted by secondary mental health services, encouraging agencies and patients to get together to draw up a care plan

Joined up working?

Statutory secondary care mental health services are characterised currently by a bewildering array of teams serving ever more specialised functions. Because of the existence of primary care gate-keeping proportionately less mental healthcare is provided in specialist settings in the UK than in most comparable countries (an exception being the Netherlands). There is a move to provide even more mental health treatment within primary care (see Chapter 3). Boundaries between primary and secondary care for mental health are also becoming less rigid, with the expectation that both primary and specialist secondary care services play an active part in the patient's management (or metaphorical 'journey').

In the UK, the NHS Plan has required statutory mental health and social care providers to form integrated services. As a result it is no longer possible to refer a patient with mental illness and social problems – for example, around housing or benefits – to a social worker. Mental health social workers now work alongside other mental health professionals in the various community and residential services, with some sharing of responsibilities between team members.

ABC of Mental Health, 2nd edition. Edited by T. Davies and T. Craig.
© 2009 Blackwell Publishing, ISBN: 978-0-7279-1639-6.

There is also a wealth of specialist private and voluntary sector provision for patients with mental health problems, offering psychotherapy, general adult psychiatry and specialist care. Service commissioners have developed service level agreements with non-statutory providers in their locality, including them in their plans for service provision for the local population as well as engaging in 'spot-purchasing'. Much day care and vocational provision is located in the voluntary sector. The bulk of supported housing and residential and nursing home places and an increasing number of long-stay hospital beds are also located in the non-statutory sector to form a 'virtual asylum' that has replaced the traditional mental hospital.

A (very) short history of mental health services

Three hundred years ago there was almost no organised provision for mentally ill patients in the UK, with the burden of care falling onto families or paid carers. For the indigent the Poor Law could offer outdoor relief, whereas disturbed patients were kept in Bridewells, gaols and workhouses. During the eighteenth century an array of lunatic hospitals, madhouses and asylums developed to treat patients with a mental illness and house those who were deemed incurable.

The early asylum doctors used the force of their personality, ineffective physical remedies and mechanical restraint to 'treat' their charges. At the Retreat in York, William Tuke (not a doctor) introduced a regimen of kindness and activity within a caring community, with minimal coercion, in the belief that this would lead to recovery. 'Moral treatment' in a small purpose-built asylum became the paradigm for care of the mentally ill and Tuke demonstrated impressive rates of discharge. Some of the important stages leading to community care are listed in Box 6.1.

Mental hospital bed numbers in England and Wales reached a peak in 1954. The subsequent decline came as the result of a complex changing environment: new medical treatments, a change in professional attitudes to include social aspects of care and more public acceptance of the mentally ill, as well as the rise of the district general hospital with its attached psychiatric unit. A series of scandals further undermined confidence in the mental hospitals. Subsequent government policy has emphasised the provision of care in non-institutional settings. Although hospital closure programmes allowed their former long-stay residents to move into a wide range of supported accommodation, effective community services for those who had never been institutionalised were slow to develop. There was persistent evidence among cohorts of patients with schizophrenia from the 1960s to the 1990s of family burden, poor quality discharge planning, lack of follow-up and a dearth of practical help for patients and carers.

Community care reforms set out by the UK Department of Health introduced parallel systems of care run by health and social services, the Care Programme Approach (CPA) and case management, the latter a mechanism for purchasing social care. During the 1990s, services adopted the model of the community mental health team (CMHT): a multidisciplinary team responsible for providing comprehensive care to adults within a defined catchment area. The murder of Jonathan Zito by Christopher Clunis in 1992 and the subsequent inquiry added to public concern over the perceived risks of care in the community and prompted a greater emphasis on risk management.

A brief account of contemporary mental health policy

The arrival of New Labour in 1997 led to a further raft of policy initiatives on mental health services (relevant policy documents are available at www.nimhe.org.uk). The National Service Framework (NSF) for Mental Health set out a vision for mental healthcare in England and Wales that spanned prevention, primary care and secondary and specialist services. Subsequently, the NHS Plan required local health economies to set up a range of specialist 'functional' teams to complement the generic CMHTs (Box 6.2).

The vision in the NSF for Mental Health and the NHS Plan was for services to treat patients with dignity, to listen to their views and to respect the role and skills of carers. There is a requirement to include patients at every level in the development and delivery of mental health services. Carers must also be offered an assessment of their own needs and a written care plan. The NHS Plan required the appointment of carer support workers, strengthening carer support networks and more respite care to be available.

Other policy developments have set standards for psychiatric intensive care and acute inpatient care, emphasised the needs of women and people from ethnic minorities, and recommended the development of specific personality disorder services.

Initiatives to promote integrated care

Care Programme Approach (CPA)

Since its introduction in 1991, mental health services have used the CPA as the framework for the care of everyone accepted by secondary mental health services. There are two levels of the CPA, standard and enhanced. Mental health professionals should take into account the needs for health and social care of the patient (and his or her carer) in agreeing the level of CPA. Some form of risk assessment is also mandatory. Patients placed on enhanced CPA should have a named care coordinator and be in receipt of a multidisciplinary care package that is defined by a written care plan (copied to the patient) and reviewed regularly. The Care Programme Approach reviews provide a forum for agencies and patients to get together to review the care plan. Those on standard CPA see just one mental health professional and have a more straightforward care plan.

It is becoming the norm for CPA documentation to be held on an electronic care record that is accessible (with appropriate safeguards) throughout a local service system. Once mental health services accept a patient, the care coordinator should keep primary care informed about their progress by, for example, inviting the GP to come to the regular CPA reviews. In practice, this sharing of care has not worked well.

Working with primary care: challenges and solutions

Shared care is a term to describe a team approach to care, with professionals from primary and secondary care contributing to a patient's care package in a coordinated way. Barriers to shared care include the negative stereotyping of patients with mental illness – whom primary care staff may consider as 'difficult' and causing extra work – and the lack of relevant expertise within primary care. Staff in secondary services often lack understanding of how primary care works and have unrealistic expectations of what can be provided within primary care.

Many GPs have direct access to psychologists and counsellors who work in the practice. A number of additional initiatives have been introduced by the NSF for Mental Health to improve both the capacity of primary care to treat mental disorders and joint working between primary and secondary care (Box 6.3). Link-working, which is facilitated when each practice relates to a single CMHT, can allow ready exchange of information about patients and service developments such as a practice register for severe mental illness.

There is also an emerging role for the GP with a special interest in mental health. The GMS contract for GPs, introduced in 2004, has five mental health targets, achievement of which is remunerated. Although these targets do not focus on the bulk of the mental health morbidity experienced in primary care, they do encourage communication with secondary care and reward primary care for managing the physical health needs of patients with severe mental illness. As yet, none of these initiatives has been subject to rigorous formal evaluation.

Patient-held records

To foster working in partnership with patients for both primary and secondary care services, there have been pilot studies looking at the use of patient-held records. Patients appreciate having them, and they improve communication across the primary–secondary care interface but information on their impact is again limited.

NICE guidelines and mental health care

NICE guidelines (available at www.nice.org.uk) are evidence-based statements of best practice. They are set to change further the delivery of mental health treatment, and, in particular, the balance between primary and secondary care. The NICE schizophrenia guideline underlines the importance of primary care in the detection of onset of psychosis and in the monitoring of the physical health of patients with established illness. The depression and anxiety guidelines indicate a shift in the balance of service provision towards primary care, adopting a 'stepped care' model, with a wider range of interventions being available in primary care. General practitioners and other front-line medical professionals are given a key role in the NICE self-harm guideline. The implementation of NICE guidelines, which tend to emphasise the efficacy of psychological approaches to treatment, represents a formidable challenge to both primary and secondary care.

The role of secondary care mental health services

Defining thresholds of need

Primary care – including GPs, practice nurses and attached mental health staff – manages the vast majority of patients with mental health problems. Only a small proportion of patients are referred to secondary care, although referral patterns are highly variable between GPs; one aim of primary care protocols is to ensure a degree of uniformity in the threshold for referral onto secondary care (Box 6.4).

Patients in contact with secondary care have characteristics that are relatively uncommon in primary care (Box 6.5).

Not all referrals to secondary mental heath services come from primary care. Arrangements for direct patient access vary, although CMHTs must respond to requests for assessments under the Mental Health Act and generally they have links with local housing providers. Occasionally hospital specialists make referrals, particularly to psychiatric liaison services (see Chapter 4). Regrettably a significant proportion of the more severely ill patients present in crisis to accident and emergency departments, via the police or the courts.

What do specialist mental health services do?

Secondary mental health services seek to meet both the specific mental health and ordinary human needs of their patients (Figure 6.1). In order to do this they must undertake a number of functions (Box 6.6).

Given the complex problems that patients with severe mental illnesses experience, to be effective community mental health services must work flexibly with a range of people and organisations (Box 6.7).

What makes up a contemporary adult mental health service?

Specialist mental health services in the UK provide care for a defined population that is commissioned in accordance with central guidance by the responsible Primary Care Trust and Social Services Authority. In addition to the plethora of community teams required by policy and inpatient facilities, a local secondary service comprises many other teams and settings. For example, there are 30 separate teams operating within the London Borough of Croydon Integrated Adult Mental Health Service (CIAMHS; Box 6.8).

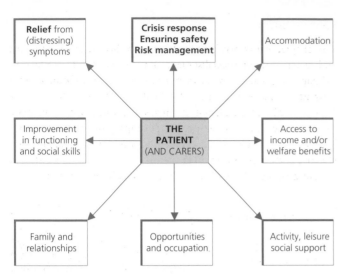

Figure 6.1 Needs of patients with a mental illness: an illustration. Needs in bold are specific to patients with a mental illness and will be provided by mental health services. Other needs are common to everyone but patients with severe mental illness may require additional support to meet them.

Box 6.6 **Functions of a specialist community mental health service**

- Assessment of mental health needs
- Crisis management
- Managing risky behaviours
- Acute interventions and treatments
- Longer term interventions and treatments
- Long-term support and care

Box 6.7 **Community mental health services work with a range of people and organisations**

- Patients with mental health needs, sometimes seen with their parents, partners or families
- Carers, families and others involved in providing care
- Specialised counselling, psychology and psychotherapy services
- Voluntary sector and private mental health service providers
- Social care providers with links to housing, benefits and employment agencies
- Criminal justice system, police, probation, courts and prisons

---

These teams are supplemented by local independent sector provision, including advocacy, psychotherapeutic, residential and day care services. In addition, CIAMHS makes regular use of tertiary services that have specific expertise not available locally, most commonly provision for the assessment and treatment of eating disorders, neuropsychiatry and comorbid autistic spectrum disorder. Some patients with particularly difficult problems and specialist needs might need to be placed in purchased NHS and independent sector out-of-area provision.

Box 6.8 **Teams operating within the Croydon Integrated Adult Mental Health Service (CIAMHS)**

Residential services
- Acute ward x 3
- Psychiatric intensive care ward
- Women's (residential) unit
- Post-discharge hostel*
- Crisis residential unit*
- Rehabilitation ward
- Homelessness Assessment Unit*

Community teams
- Community mental health team x 8
- Assertive outreach team
- Rehabilitation, recovery and continuing care team
- Early onset psychosis team
- Crisis resolution/home treatment team
- Mother and baby team

Other services
- Psychological therapies service
- Primary care counselling service
- Psychotherapy service
- Therapeutic intervention service
- Liaison service
- Day care service
- Telephone helpline
- Psychosexual clinic

CIAMHS is under one management structure but funded from both health and social care budgets (and the Supporting People funding stream*). It includes both health and social care teams: all the core community teams are fully integrated

Challenges to using specialist mental health services

Accessing services

In the past, when the CMHT was the sole focus of secondary care, access routes were relatively simple. The current functionally differentiated model of mental health services offers a potentially bewildering range of options for referrers, patients and carers. Localities vary as to their access routes, with the majority providing access for new referrals within working hours via the CMHT. Although the CMHT is the usual point of first contact, direct referral may be possible to some services, such as the local psychology or psychotherapy department and certain specialist services where the primary care diagnosis is known to be reliable, such as eating disorder and mother-and-baby services. In a few services, direct referral of suspected new cases of psychosis to an early intervention team is possible. Once patients have been assessed and the mental health service takes on their care, they come automatically under the CPA.

Responding to crises

Patients, carers and referrers regularly complain about the difficulties they experience in accessing mental health services in a crisis. During working hours, the local CMHT is usually the first point of contact. Out of hours access may be through helplines and the local

---

Box 6.9 **Initial management plan for a patient in crisis**

This may include
- Advice for the referrer on how to manage the patient
- Immediate treatment
- Referral onto another agency, for example, in the voluntary sector
- Referral onto another community team that will put together a comprehensive care plan for the immediate period and consider longer term needs as appropriate
- Admission to inpatient care, including compulsory admission under mental health legislation

---

accident and emergency department. Approved social workers and Section 12 approved doctors should always be available to undertake Mental Health Act assessments. In some areas, the Crisis Resolution Team (CRT)/Home Treatment Team (HTT) offers direct access to all patients in a self-defined crisis or at the request of primary care, although there is evidence that CRT/HTTs are only effective at reducing hospital admissions when assessing and treating patients at the point of admission to hospital.

Whatever its provenance, any element of the specialist mental health services responding to a crisis should undertake an assessment and make a formulation, including an initial management plan (Box 6.9).

Some of the functional teams provide 24-hour cover, and, therefore, arrangements for known patients in crisis vary. They should be specified within the CPA documentation as the contingency and crisis plan.

Conclusion

This chapter gives a brief introduction to the historical development and current status of specialist mental health services. The move from primarily hospital-based to community-based care has brought with it significant benefits in terms of patient care. However, the increasing complexity of the mental health system, which is set to increase further as the patient choice agenda develops, poses significant challenges to primary and secondary care services as they seek to provide effective and seamless care. In the future, electronic care records and patient-held records may help make this laudable goal a reality.

Further information

www.nimhe.org.uk
www.nice.org.uk

Further reading

Appleby L. *The National Service Framework for Mental Health – Five years on.* Department of Health, London, 2004.

Burns T. *Community mental health teams. A guide to current practices.* Oxford University Press, Oxford, 2004.

Department of Health. *National Service Framework for Mental Health.* DH, London, 1999.

Mynors-Wallis L, Moore M, Maguire J, Hollingbery T. *Shared care in mental health.* Oxford University Press, Oxford, 2002.

Rose N. Historical changes in mental health practice. In: Thornicroft G, Szmukler G, eds. *Textbook of community psychiatry.* Oxford University Press, Oxford, 2001: 12–27.

CHAPTER 7

Anxiety

Stirling Moorey and Anthony S Hale

OVERVIEW

- Anxiety is a common but unpleasant experience that might be a normal reaction to circumstances but can become chronic, self-perpetuating and debilitating
- Anxiety disorders should be differentiated from each other, and from other reactions to stress, as their optimal treatments differ
- Self-help manuals or patient support groups assist many patients in overcoming their anxiety without recourse to specialist treatments
- Psychological intervention (e.g. cognitive behavioural therapy, CBT) is indicated for most moderately severe anxiety disorders, alone or in combination with medication

---

Box 7.1 **Anxiety disorders should be differentiated from other reactions to stress**

- Anxiety is a prominent feature of reactions to stress
- **Acute stress reaction:** a rapid response (in minutes or hours) to sudden or unforeseen stressful life events, leading to anxiety with autonomic arousal and some disorientation
- **Adjustment reactions:** slower responses that occur days or weeks after life events (such as loss of job, moving house or divorce) with symptoms of anxiety, irritability and depression (without biological symptoms). These are generally self-limiting and are helped by reassurance, 'ventilation' of feelings and problem solving
- **Post-traumatic stress disorder:** a more profound stress reaction

---

Anxiety is an unpleasant emotional state characterised by fearfulness and unwanted and distressing physical symptoms. It is a normal and appropriate response to stress but becomes pathological when it is disproportionate to the severity of the stress, continues after the stressor has gone or occurs in the absence of any external stressor (Box 7.1). Neurotic disorders with anxiety as a prominent symptom are common. A recent survey of UK households by the Office of National Statistics found that one in six of all adults met the criteria for a neurotic disorder in the week before the survey. The commonest diagnosis was mixed anxiety and depression (9%), followed by generalised anxiety disorder (4%). The remaining disorders (depression, phobias, obsessive–compulsive disorder (OCD) and panic) ranged from 3% to 1%. Anxiety disorders are often chronic and can have a disabling effect on the sufferer and his or her family.

Although there is considerable overlap between the various anxiety disorders, it is important to make a diagnosis as they have different optimal treatments (Table 7.1)

The National Institute for Health and Clinical Excellence (NICE; www.nice.org.uk) has produced evidence-based guidelines that emphasise the importance of providing treatment for anxiety in primary care where possible and referring on to secondary care if initial treatment is not effective. They highlight the strong evidence base for cognitive behavioural therapy (CBT).

In a basic cognitive model of anxiety, anxiety is defined as a normal reaction to perceived threat or danger. In anxiety disorders, there is a distorted interpretation of the threat that is faced: the likelihood of harm is exaggerated, and the consequences of the harm overestimated, whereas the chances of rescue are underestimated. Someone with a dog phobia will overestimate their chances of encountering a dog in a given situation, will catastrophise about the likelihood of being attacked, and will underestimate their chances of dealing with the situation effectively. The response to the perceived threat is often avoidance, which tends to reinforce the belief that a given situation is dangerous.

Specific cognitive behavioural models (Box 7.2) and therapies have been developed for each of the anxiety disorders, all based on this basic model of anxiety. Cognitive behavioural therapy involves a combination of verbal discussion and questioning of beliefs plus very practical behavioural experiments to test the anxious beliefs. Many practitioners also use more behavioural techniques of graded exposure to feared situations, particularly with specific phobias and OCD.

Generalised anxiety disorder

Generalised anxiety disorder (GAD) affects 4% of the general population, with a slight female preponderance, but accounts for almost 30% of 'psychiatric' consultations in general practice. Its onset is usually in early adulthood and its course may be chronic,

---

ABC of Mental Health, 2nd edition. Edited by T. Davies and T. Craig.
©2009 Blackwell Publishing, ISBN: 978-0-7279-1639-6.

Table 7.1 Summary of treatment options for the anxiety disorders

Anxiety disorder	Pharmacotherapy	Psychological therapy
Generalised anxiety disorder Acute anxiety	Benzodiazepines (should not usually be used beyond two to four weeks) Sedating antihistamines	
Generalised anxiety disorder Chronic anxiety	*First line* Selective serotonin reuptake inhibitors (SSRIs) should be the first choice *Second line* Tricyclics (not addictive but many side effects) Buspirone (delayed onset but no dependence) β-blockers (block peripheral manifestations of anxiety, especially cardiac) *Treatment-resistant cases* Switch to or combine with psychological therapy	*First line* Cognitive behavioural therapy (CBT) Self-help CBT *Second line (for cases with major interpersonal difficulties)* Counselling Psychodynamic psychotherapy *Treatment-resistant cases* Switch to or combine with pharmacotherapy
Panic disorder and agoraphobia	*First line* SSRIs (may exacerbate anxiety initially) Benzodiazepines should not be used in panic disorder *Second line* Tricyclic antidepressants (imipramine or clomipramine) *Treatment-resistant cases* Switch to or combine with psychological therapy	*First line* CBT Self-help CBT *Treatment-resistant cases* Switch to or combine with pharmacotherapy
Social phobia	*First line* SSRIs *Second line* Monoamine oxidase inhibitors (MAOIs) (probably best initiated by mental health specialist) β-blockers used occasionally for somatic symptoms of performance anxiety *Treatment-resistant cases* Venlafaxine, clonazepam, valproate	*First line* CBT *Treatment-resistant cases* Switch to or combine with pharmacotherapy
Specific phobia	Medication ineffective	*First line* CBT (*in vivo* exposure)
Post-traumatic stress disorder (PTSD)	Medication should not be first-line treatment for PTSD unless the patient prefers not to have a psychological treatment or severity of depression precludes him or her from psychological treatment *Second line* Paroxetine or mirtazapine (general practice) Amitriptyline (secondary care) *Treatment-resistant cases* Phenelzine (secondary care)	*First line* CBT Eye movement desensitisation reprocessing (EMDR) *Second line* Psychodynamic psychotherapy (if not suitable for CBT and evidence of early childhood trauma) *Treatment-resistant cases* Add or switch to pharmacotherapy
Obsessive–compulsive disorder	*First line* SSRIs (fluoxetine, paroxetine, sertraline and citalopram) Clomipramine *Treatment-resistant cases* Quetiapine or risperidone augmentation of antidepressants (specialist centres)	*First line* CBT including exposure with response prevention *Treatment-resistant cases* CBT plus medication Inpatient CBT

Box 7.2 **Cognitive models of anxiety disorders**

Disorder	Focus of attention	Perceived threat
Panic	Autonomic symptoms	Impending internal disaster
Social phobia	Internal impression of self as social object	Negative social evaluation
Obsessive–compulsive disorder	Intrusive thoughts	Responsibility for harm to self or others
Post-traumatic stress disorder	Trauma or its consequences	Serious continuing threat to self or the world
Generalised anxiety disorder	Wide variety of situations and worry itself	Danger to self or others

with a worse prognosis in women. Some genetic predisposition is present, childhood traumas such as separations may confer vulnerability, and it may be triggered and maintained by stressful life events.

It is characterised by irrational worries, motor tension, hyper-vigilance and somatic symptoms (Box 7.3). For most sufferers it tends to be mild, but in severe cases it may be very disabling.

Management

NICE guidelines recommend psychological therapy (CBT), medication (selective serotonin reuptake inhibitors, SSRIs) and self-help. These should be delivered in primary care where possible. If the patient does not respond to two of these treatment options, then referral for specialist assessment and treatment is indicated.

> **Box 7.3 Diagnosis of generalised anxiety disorder**
>
> - Persistent (>six months) 'free floating' anxiety or apprehension
> - Disturbed sleep (early and middle insomnia, not restful)
> - Muscle tension, tremor, restlessness
> - Autonomic overactivity (sweating, tachycardia, epigastric discomfort)
> - May be secondary to or subsumed by other psychiatric disorders such as depression or schizophrenia (see Chapter 1)
> - Exclude physical disorders that may mimic anxiety:
>   - Excessive caffeine use
>   - Thyrotoxicosis, parathyroid disease
>   - Hypoglycaemia
>   - Drug or alcohol withdrawal
>   - Phaeochromocytoma, carcinoid syndrome
>   - Cardiac dysrhythmias, mitral valve disease

Self-help and general management

This may be the first line of treatment for less severe cases, and can be used in conjunction with medication. General support and information about the condition with an empathic understanding of the life circumstances that may be contributing to the anxiety can be helpful. Information about local self-help groups that can offer face-to-face meetings or sometimes telephone conferences should be given. Self-help books based on cognitive behavioural principles can be made available in GP surgeries. Computerised CBT has also been shown to be effective in GAD. Other self-help activities such as exercise and fitness programmes may have an anxiolytic effect.

Drug treatment

Benzodiazepines

Acute GAD can be treated with benzodiazepines. Onset of action is fast, but tolerance develops with chronic use; this leads to increased dosage with acute withdrawal reactions on cessation in 30% of cases and chronic reactions in 10%. Side effects include sedation and amnesia and possibly also anxiety and depression: there is substantial potential for misuse and an interaction with alcohol. Benzodiazepines should not be used beyond four weeks. Sedating antihistamines may also be used in acute anxiety.

Selective serotonin reuptake inhibitors

More chronic conditions are best treated with antidepressants. A SSRI is the antidepressant of choice, usually starting at half the dose used to treat depression and increased as appropriate. Anxiety symptoms may be exacerbated in the first week of treatment and the response is usually seen within six weeks, increasing further with time. If there is no response after a 12-week course, another SSRI or another form of therapy should be offered. Once an optimal dose is reached treatment should continue for at least six months. To minimise the risk of discontinuation symptoms when stopping, SSRIs should be withdrawn gradually.

Tricyclic antidepressants

The side effects of tricyclic antidepressants make them an unnecessary choice as first-line treatment for anxiety disorders.

Buspirone

Although dependence has not been seen with buspirone, many patients are dubious about its efficacy, perhaps because of its slow onset of action. For chronic anxiety, this is not such a drawback. A trial of up to eight weeks' treatment with at least 30 mg buspirone daily, after gradually increasing the dose for the first two weeks, is often successful.

β-blockers

These may be helpful in patients with marked somatic symptoms, particularly tachycardia.

> Some patients – especially those with chronic anxiety, a tendency to self-treat with alcohol and a long history of benzodiazepine use – are difficult to manage except with benzodiazepines. When benzodiazepines are used, those with a slower onset of action (not the same as half-life), such as the GABA partial-agonist clonazepam, may cause less dependence and withdrawal symptoms than diazepam or lorazepam

Psychological therapy

The availability of psychological therapy in primary care settings varies considerably. NICE guidelines explicitly recommend cognitive behaviour therapy delivered by suitably trained and supervised therapists who can demonstrate they adhere closely to empirically grounded treatment protocols. In many practices medication and self-help will be the first treatments for GAD, with referral to a specialist psychological therapies service if these are not effective. Where CBT is used in primary care it may be short term (8–10 hours), and is then best integrated with structured self-help materials the patient can use between sessions to maximise the impact of therapy.

Cognitive behavioural therapy for generalised anxiety uses techniques to reduce the pervasive appraisal of threat (testing negative predictions through discussion and experiments), overcome avoidance (behavioural experiments and exposure), manage worry (scheduling worry time) and cope with anxiety symptoms (relaxation). The NICE guidelines do not support the use of counselling or psychodynamic therapy in GAD. However, in some cases where there are significant interpersonal difficulties or comorbidity with personality problems, these less structured therapies may have a place.

Panic disorder with or without agoraphobia

Panic attacks may occur as part of several conditions. However, panic disorder is characterised by unpredictable attacks of severe anxiety with pronounced autonomic symptoms not related to any particular situation. Common features are shortness of breath, fear of dying or of going crazy, and an urgent desire to flee regardless of the consequences (Box 7.4).

One-year prevalence of panic disorder is 1–2%, with a lifetime prevalence of 1.5–3.5%. Onset is commonest in adolescents or in

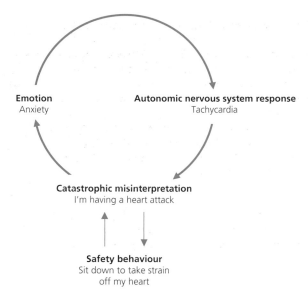

Figure 7.1 Vicious circle in panic disorder.

people in their mid-30s, whereas onset after 45 is rare. The course of the disorder is variable: sometimes chronic but waxing and waning in severity, or rarely it may be episodic (Box 7.5). There is evidence of genetic transmission, with first-degree relatives of patients at four to seven times greater risk than the general population.

Agoraphobia is characterised by a fear of being in places or situations from which escape might be difficult or rescue unavailable. Agoraphobics are commonly afraid of being away from home, travelling by car, train or tube, using lifts or being in a crowd of people. The majority, though not all, of people with agoraphobia will also have had spontaneous panic attacks.

Management

NICE guidelines recommend psychological therapy (CBT), medication (SSRIs) and self-help. These should be delivered in primary care where possible. If the patient does not respond to two of these treatment options, then referral for specialist assessment and treatment is indicated.

Self-help and general management

As with GAD, general support and information about the condition with an understanding of how the panics might arise in the setting of life stress can be helpful. For some patients an early explanation of the cognitive model of panic – how a catastrophic misinterpretation of normal autonomic symptoms (tachycardia, palpitations, breathlessness, dizziness) as signs of heart attack, collapse or impending death leads to increased anxiety and further symptoms (Figure 7.1) – can help them to reattribute the

terrifying feelings to anxiety. This may be enough to prevent the panic attacks from becoming chronic. In more established cases, information about local self-help groups that use behavioural principles can give support and practical guidance. Self-help books and computerised CBT also have a role.

Drug treatment

NICE guidelines discourage the prescription of benzodiazepines in panic because they are associated with poorer long-term outcome. Sedating antihistamines and antipsychotics are also contraindicated. Both tricyclic antidepressants and SSRIs have been shown to be effective for panic, but the latter are preferred because of their relative lack of side effects. Selective serotonin reuptake inhibitors are initiated at low doses and the dose increased until a therapeutic response is achieved. If there is no effect after 12 weeks, a tricyclic (imipramine or clomipramine) may be tried. When successful, treatment should be continued for six months. Antidepressants often produce an initial increase in anxiety in the first few weeks of treatment before therapeutic benefits appear, leading to poor compliance. This may be overcome by explanation, starting with a low dose with slow increase to therapeutic dose.

Psychological treatment

Cognitive behavioural therapy is the treatment of choice. Cognitive therapy for panic in primary care can be effective in six to eight sessions. Treatment focuses on helping patients test their catastrophic fears about the physical symptoms of anxiety. For instance, if a patient feels faint and fears she will collapse, the therapist may test this with her by conducting a behavioural experiment: therapist and patient both over-breathe in the session and then stand up to find out if they will actually collapse. The patient discovers that although she feels dizzy she does not fall in the way she fears. An important part of this process is identifying the subtle forms of avoidance or safety behaviours the patient uses (e.g. holding on to furniture when feeling faint, opening windows when feeling unable to breathe) and getting her to give them up.

For some patients the fear of having panic attacks can lead to the avoidance of certain situations associated with panic. These are often places where the patient feels unable to access help. Testing these fears through exposure to the avoided situation, usually in a controlled and graded way is a highly effective treatment for agoraphobia. The patient draws up a hierarchy of situations and practises entering the situations as homework, sometimes with the assistance of a friend or family member as a co-therapist. As he or she becomes confident in a situation they move on to the next step of the hierarchy and eventually carry out experiments alone, without the support of their co-therapist.

Social phobia

Social phobia is a persistent fear of performing in social situations, especially where strangers are present or where the person fears embarrassment (Box 7.6). Patients fear that others will think them stupid, weak or crazy, and exposure to the feared situation provokes an immediate anxiety attack. Patients recognise that their fear is excessive, but their anxiety and avoidance behaviour may interfere markedly with their daily routine, work or social life. Blushing is common, and patients may avoid eating, drinking or writing in public.

There is some genetic predisposition, onset may follow a particular stressful or embarrassing experience, or be insidious, and the disorder usually follows a chronic course. Symptoms often start in adolescence or even childhood, and may be associated with poor social or academic performance. The incidence of social phobia is about 2%, but lifetime prevalence ranges from 3% to 13%. In some community studies social phobia is more common in women than men, but the sexes are equally represented in clinical samples. Alcohol is used by many people as a coping strategy. Assessment should include a drinking history.

Management
Drug treatment
Selective serotonin reuptake inhibitors are the first-line pharmacological treatment. Monoamine oxidase inhibitors (MAOIs; phenelzine or moclobemide) are the second line of treatment. Moclobemide is probably the drug of choice, but high doses may be required and treatment should continue for a minimum of three months.

> **Box 7.6 Social phobias – diagnosis**
>
> - Extreme, persistent fear of social situations
> - Fear of humiliation or embarrassment
> - Exposure provokes extreme anxiety
> - Fear recognised as excessive or unreasonable
> - Avoidance of situations
> - Anxious anticipation
> Look out for accompanying alcohol problems

Psychological treatment
Cognitive behavioural therapy has proven efficacy in social phobia. Paradoxically, this does not focus on external threat but on the internal image of how the patient thinks he looks to others. Treatments combining imaginary and actual exposure produce modest gains but seem as effective as more complex regimens. Cognitive behavioural therapy is promising, either alone or in combination with an antidepressant, but seems most effective in the third of cases with circumscribed social phobias.

Specific (isolated) phobias

These are circumscribed fears of specific objects or situations. Some community samples have shown an annual prevalence as high as 9% in the general population. Most phobias start in childhood, but situational phobias have a second peak of onset among people in their middle 20s. Particular types of phobias seem to aggregate in families, with some evidence of biological predisposition. Other predisposing factors include traumatic events that affected the patient or were observed in others, and repeated warnings from others about situations. Phobias that persist into adult life usually have a chronic course (Box 7.7).

Management
Successful treatment is almost exclusively with behavioural therapy. Drugs are of little use.

Post-traumatic stress disorder

Anxiety and other symptoms may follow a severe trauma such as an assault or a serious accident. About a quarter of people will go on to develop post-traumatic stress disorder (PTSD) (Box 7.8). The most distressing symptom is often the presence of re-experiencing symptoms such as flashbacks and nightmares of the traumatic event. There is avoidance of situations or people who remind the victim of the event and a pervasive hyperarousal and hypervigilance to possible danger. It is as if the circumstances of the trauma, although past, are still actively present, thus putting the person in continued danger. There may also be significant emotional numbing. There is considerable comorbidity with depression,

> **Box 7.7 Specific (isolated) phobias – diagnosis**
>
> - Extreme, persistent and unreasonable fear
> - Cued by appearance or anticipation of specific object or situation
> - Specific objects include
>   - Animals (spiders, snakes)
>   - Natural environment (heights, water, storms)
>   - Blood, injections, injury (may provoke particularly strong vasovagal response with fainting)
>   - Specific situations (driving, flying, tunnels, lifts, bridges, rivers, enclosed spaces)
> - Avoidance of situation often with secondary fear of the phobia itself (phobophobia)

Box 7.8 **Post-traumatic stress disorder – diagnosis**

- Exceptional stressor
- Intrusive flashbacks, vivid memories, recurring dreams
- Emotional numbness, detachment initially
- Distress on re-exposure, leading to avoidance of similar circumstances
- Hypervigilance and hyperarousal
- Psychogenic amnesia, insomnia, irritability, anger, poor concentration, distractible, diminished interests, pessimistic mood

Severity affected by

- Premorbid mental or psychological problems
- Repeated similar stress
- Human agency – more severe if stressor caused by another person

anxiety states and other psychosomatic syndromes. If patients present with some of the key symptoms of PTSD, or unexplained physical symptoms, a sensitive enquiry should be made about whether they have experienced a recent or more distant trauma.

Self-help and general management

Debriefing after a trauma should not be offered routinely as it is ineffective and may even be harmful. Symptoms remit with time in the majority of people. When symptoms are mild and have been present for less than four weeks, 'watchful waiting' with follow-up in a month is recommended. Information for patients, family and carers should be available to help them understand the nature of their reactions and their time course. If available, brief CBT (eight to ten sessions) may be helpful in the first three months for more severe PTSD. In PTSD that persists beyond three months, a course of CBT or eye movement desensitisation reprocessing (EMDR) is recommended. This will normally be provided on an outpatient basis.

Drug treatment

NICE guidelines recommend that drug treatment should not be the first line of treatment for PTSD. Indications for the use of medication are:

- Depression where the severity of symptoms or risk of suicide precludes the use of psychological therapy. Less severe depression usually responds when the PTSD is treated
- Insomnia in the early stages of PTSD where short-term use of hypnotics can be helpful
- Preference not to engage in a psychological treatment for PTSD
- Failure to respond to adequate trial of trauma-focused psychological treatment.

Paroxetine and mirtazapine are recommended as the drug treatment of choice for PTSD in primary care. NICE recommends that amitriptyline and phenelzine are used only by mental health specialists. As with other anxiety disorders, treatment may need to start at a lower dose. Response is usually seen within eight weeks, but may take 12 weeks. Treatment should be continued for at least 12 months, followed by gradual withdrawal.

Psychological treatment

Cognitive behavioural therapy and EMDR are the two treatments recommended by NICE.

Cognitive behavioural therapy involves techniques to help patients reprocess their memories of the trauma, to overcome the associated avoidance and to rebuild their lives. Reprocessing can take the form of exposure in imagination to the memories of the event, retelling the story through talking or writing, and examining the memories for unhelpful distorted interpretations. Reprocessing helps patients to integrate memories into their general memory system so they are not separated off as fragmented elements that are experienced as distressing intrusions. Avoidance can be dealt with by setting up behavioural experiments to test whether feared situations are as frightening as they seem. Cognitive techniques can help patients deal with the way the event has challenged their fundamental views of themselves and their world.

Eye movement desensitisation reprocessing involves accessing the thoughts, feelings and imagery associated with the trauma while engaging in repeated, rhythmic side-to-side movements of the eyes. This appears to be a rapid form of desensitisation to the trauma. The process is then repeated, replacing the negative cognitions with positive ones. Treatment lasts for 10 to 12 sessions. Eye movement desensitisation reprocessing has been shown to be effective in randomised controlled trials.

Patients who have complex PTSD associated with prolonged abusive experiences in childhood often have comorbid personality difficulties. Trauma-focused therapy may need to be followed by longer term psychodynamic therapy; in some cases it may be difficult for patients to engage in a structured, focused therapy and psychodynamic psychotherapy may be the best treatment option.

Obsessive–compulsive disorder

Obsessions are intrusive thoughts, images or urges that are recognised by the individual to be irrational and unwanted and are usually resisted (the resistance diminishes with chronicity). They may be fears that the person might harm someone or might inadvertently contaminate or infect someone. Although everyone experiences intrusions, the person with OCD tends to assume an excessive responsibility for them, concluding that they might be capable of causing harm or might be morally reprehensible because they have them. Compulsions are repetitive behaviours or mental acts that the person feels driven to perform. They are often carried out in order to avoid or neutralise the feared consequence of an obsession. For instance, someone with a fear that he might accidentally pass on germs to his children might engage in frequent and excessive hand washing. Checking and cleaning rituals are the most common manifestations.

Obsessive–compulsive disorder has a lifetime prevalence of 2% with an equal sex distribution. Onset is in adolescence or early adulthood, but treatment may not be sought until 10 or 15 years after the symptoms begin (Box 7.9).

Box 7.9 **Screening questions for obsessive–compulsive disorder (from NICE guidelines for OCD)**

- Do you wash or clean a lot?
- Do you check things a lot?
- Is there any thought that keeps bothering you that you'd like to get rid of but can't?
- Do your daily activities take a long time to finish?
- Are you concerned about putting things in a special order or are you very upset by mess?
- Do these problems trouble you?

Drug treatment

The selective serotonin reuptake inhibitors fluoxetine, fluvoxamine, paroxetine, sertraline and citalopram have been shown to be effective in treatment of OCD. Treatment should begin at a standard dose but if the response is inadequate, and there are no significant side effects, a gradual increase in dose should be considered after four to six weeks. Response is slower than in depression and some patients with OCD may need higher doses for therapeutic effect (e.g. fluoxetine 40–60 mg, paroxetine 60 mg). If treatment is effective, it should be continued for at least 12 months to prevent relapse and allow for further improvements. Continued treatment over two years halves the relapse rate.

The tricyclic antidepressant clomipramine has been shown to be effective in treatment of OCD, but has more side effects than the SSRIs. Other tricyclics should not be prescribed.

Use of other medications (e.g. augmentation with antipsychotics) should only be considered in treatment-resistant cases and restricted to mental health specialists.

Psychological treatment

Cognitive behavioural therapy is the treatment of choice for OCD. The majority of patients experience an improvement, though there are often residual symptoms. Relapse rates following the withdrawal of antidepressants are high, whereas the gains made with a course of CBT tend to be maintained over one to two year follow-up. Treatments involve some degree of exposure to the obsessions, combined with response prevention. For instance, someone with a contamination fear might touch the bottom of their shoes and refrain from washing their hands. Initially their anxiety would be raised considerably, but over the course of an exposure session this would reduce to manageable levels. Some of this work is done with the therapist but patients are also expected to carry out self-exposure work at home.

Personal accounts of mental health problems

Drake S. *A cry for help*. Chipmunkapublishing, Brentwood, Essex, 2006. www.chipmunka.com

Further information

Information about anxiety and panic attacks, agoraphobia, PTSD, obsessive–compulsive disorder and social phobia can be obtained from the British Association for Behavioural and Cognitive Psychotherapy: www.babcp.org.uk.
Burns DD. *Feeling good: the new mood therapy*. Avon Books/HarperCollins, London, 2000.
Butler G. *Overcoming social anxiety and shyness*. Constable & Robinson, London, 1999.
Greenberger D & Padesky CA. *Mind over mood: Change how you feel by changing the way you think*. Guildford Press, New York, 1995.
Herbert C, Wetmore A. *Overcoming traumatic stress*. Constable & Robinson, London, 2001.
Kennerley H. *Overcoming anxiety*. Constable & Robinson, London, 1997.
Veale D, Willson R. *Overcoming obsessive–compulsive disorder*. Constable & Robinson, London, 2005.

Glaser J. *Hear the silence*. Chipmunkapublishing, Brentwood, Essex, 2006. www.chipmunka.com
Jordan RD. *Clinical depression*. Chipmunkapublishing, Brentwood, Essex, 2006. www.chipmunka.com

Further reading

Davidson JR. Pharmacotherapy of generalised anxiety disorder. *J Clin Psych* 2001; **62**: 46–50.
National Institute for Health and Clinical Excellence. *Post-traumatic stress disorder (PTSD): The management of PTSD in adults and children in primary and secondary care*. NICE guideline CG26. NICE, London, 2005. http://guidance.nice.org.uk/CG26/
National Institute for Health and Clinical Excellence. *Obsessive-compulsive disorder: Core interventions in the treatment of obsessive-compulsive disorder and body dysmorphic disorder*. NICE guideline CG31. NICE, London, 2005. http://guidance.nice.org.uk/CG31/
National Institute for Health and Clinical Excellence. *Anxiety (amended): Management of anxiety (panic disorder, with or without agoraphobia, and generalised anxiety disorder) in adults in primary, secondary and community care*. NICE guideline CG22. NICE, London, 2007. http://guidance.nice.org.uk/CG22/
Taylor D, Paton C, Kerwin R (eds). *The Maudsley prescribing guidelines*, 8th edn. Taylor & Francis, London, 2005.
Wells A. *Cognitive therapy for anxiety disorders*. Wiley, Chichester, 1995.

CHAPTER 8

Depression

Anthony S Hale and Teifion Davies

OVERVIEW

- Depression is one of the major causes of disability worldwide
- There are several forms of depressive disorder, but clear criteria exist for diagnosis (presence of specific features for at least two weeks)
- Moderate depression, sufficient to prevent normal functioning, responds to both antidepressants and cognitive behavioural therapy; severe depression may require additional antipsychotic medication
- Depressive episodes are often under-treated: too low a dose of antidepressant for too short a time, or changing drugs too frequently

Depression has a range of meanings – from a description of normal unhappiness, through persistent and pervasive ways of feeling and thinking, to psychosis. According to World Health Organization data, depression affects about 50 million people and causes about 10% of the global burden of disease worldwide, with women and economically impoverished people being affected disproportionately. By 2030, depression is projected to be the second greatest cause of years lived with disability worldwide. Textbook descriptions of depression seen in hospitals are often very different from presentations in primary care (Box 8.1).

In recent community surveys, 2% of the adult population suffered from pure depression (evenly distributed between mild, moderate and severe), but another 8% suffered from a mixture of anxiety and depression. Even patients with symptoms not severe enough to qualify for a diagnosis of either anxiety or depression alone have impaired working and social lives and many unexplained physical symptoms, leading to greater use of medical services.

Variable presentation of depression, particularly in primary care, may make recognition and diagnosis difficult (Box 8.2). Recent guidance by the National Institute for Health and Clinical Excellence (NICE) has suggested that patients with risk factors or previous history should be screened routinely using standard questions, or questionnaires such as the PHQ-9. Key practical questions relate to treatment: is any required at all and, if so, what sort, and for how long?

ABC of Mental Health, 2nd edition. Edited by T. Davies and T. Craig.
© 2009 Blackwell Publishing, ISBN: 978-0-7279-1639-6.

Box 8.1 **Depression in primary care**

- One in 20 visits to doctor are due to depression
- >100 depressed patients per general practitioner's list, but half unrecognised
- 20% develop chronic depression
- Why patients may not mention their depression:
  - Embarrassed
  - Avoid stigma
  - Somatisation
  - Avoid annoying doctor
  - Avoid lack of sympathy

Box 8.2 **Diagnostic features of depression**

Core features
- Pervasive low mood
- Loss of interest and enjoyment (anhedonia)
- Reduced energy (anergia), diminished activity

Other features
- Poor concentration and attention
- Poor self-esteem and self-confidence
- Ideas of guilt and unworthiness
- Bleak, pessimistic views of the future
- Ideas or acts of self-harm or suicide
- Disturbed sleep
- Diminished appetite.

For diagnosis of a depressive episode, at least two core features plus three others must be present for a minimum of two weeks

Forms of depression

Most depressions have triggering life events, especially in a first episode. Many patients present initially with physical symptoms (somatisation), and some may show multiple symptoms of depression in the apparent absence of low mood ('masked' depression).

Less severe depression has been awarded many labels, including neurotic depression, minor depression and reactive depression (not depression as a reaction to circumstances but when reactivity to events in the surroundings is preserved). It is now termed dysthymia, a persistent low grade condition. This may be complicated by episodes of more severe depression, resulting in 'double' depression in which resolution of the more severe syndrome is difficult to judge.

Many patients do not fit neatly into categories of either anxiety or depression, and the concept of mixed anxiety and depression is now recognised. The presence of physical symptoms indicates a somatic syndrome (so-called melancholic or endogenous depression) (Box 8.3). The value of these features in predicting response to treatment is not clear. The presence of psychotic features has major implications for treatment. Brief episodes of more severe depression are also recognised (brief recurrent depression). More prolonged recurrence is now termed 'recurrent depressive disorder' (formerly depressive illness).

Atypical depression is characterised by increased sleep and appetite, and weight gain. Agitated depression, more common in the elderly, may present with psychomotor agitation that is not accompanied by subjective anxiety.

Diagnosis

There are three main distinctions to be made. Is the depression an illness or 'normal' unhappiness? If it is an illness, is it a primary psychiatric condition or is it secondary to a physical illness, or to alcohol or other drugs? If it is a primary psychiatric illness, is it unipolar or bipolar?

Severity of depression is largely a question of number and intensity of characteristic symptoms. A few mild but persistent symptoms suggests dysthymia. More numerous or more severe symptoms suggest a depressive disorder. Psychotic symptoms (delusions, hallucinations) or depressive stupor are present only in severe depression.

Treatment

Much depressive illness of all types is successfully treated in primary care. The main reasons for referring depressed patients to secondary mental health services are that the condition is severe, failing to respond to treatment, complicated by other factors (such as personality disorder) or presents particular risks (Box 8.4). The presence of agitation has been shown to mask psychotic features. Patients with marked psychomotor retardation are also often difficult to treat in primary care.

Medication versus psychotherapy

Basic treatment for mild, moderate and severe depression is generally similar. The principal decision is whether to treat with drugs or a talking therapy. Surveys have shown that most patients in primary care settings would prefer a talking therapy, but evidence of effectiveness is limited to particular forms of psychotherapy.

In mild depression, a patient's response to antidepressants may be no better than to placebo, and bibliotherapy (using self-help manuals) or cognitive behavioural therapy (CBT) are more useful. For moderate depression, CBT and antidepressants are equally effective, and the two combined are superior to either alone. For more severe depression, antidepressant drugs are more effective. Cognitive behavioural therapy is a 'brief' focused psychotherapy requiring from six to 20 sessions, and its availability may be limited in some areas.

Drug treatment

The use of tricyclic antidepressants at doses well below those that are therapeutically effective (i.e. less than 125 mg daily imipramine equivalent) has often been reported, especially in primary care. Chopping and changing treatments before giving any one a chance to work (at least six to eight week trial) is also common.

Effective antidepressant drugs have been available since the 1950s. The choice is now between traditional tricyclic antidepressants (TCAs) and monoamine oxidase inhibitors (MAOIs), and more recent selective serotonin reuptake inhibitors (SSRIs), selective serotonin-noradrenaline reuptake inhibitors (SNRIs) and other monotherapy antidepressants (e.g. reboxetine, mirtazapine) (Box 8.5).

Newer drugs were developed 'rationally' to be more selective in their actions than the older antidepressants, and, hence, have far fewer serious side effects than the TCAs or the MAOIs. However, some older drugs – such as desipramine, maprotiline and nortriptyline – are also selective for noradrenaline reuptake blockade. The differences between drugs lie primarily in their side effects and their potential interactions with other drugs.

Side effects, in particular anticholinergic effects and weight gain, are thought to have a major effect on the frequency with which patients do not take antidepressants as prescribed. Careful clinical studies show large differences between older and newer antidepressants, with much higher non-adherence rates in patients taking the older drugs with more side effects. This merely demonstrates what is clinically obvious – that patients prefer taking drugs with fewer side effects.

Tricyclic antidepressants
Available since the 1950s, effective and cheap, but all have dose-related anticholinergic side effects that limit adherence. They produce variable degrees of sedation, and postural hypotension may cause falls. Cardiotoxicity in overdose. Lofepramine is relatively safe in overdose and almost free of anticholinergic side effects.

Selective serotonin reuptake inhibitors
Five now available (fluvoxamine, fluoxetine, paroxetine, sertraline and citalopram). All lack sedation and are free of anticholinergic effects. This improves adherence but gives less immediate benefit for disturbed sleep (hence, may be combined initially with low doses of sedative antidepressants or hypnotics). All seem safe in overdose. A major benefit with several is that a single or narrow range of doses can be advocated for most patients, usually taken once daily, overcoming the tendency in general practice to prescribe doses of a third to a half of effective therapeutic dose.

Monoamine oxidase inhibitors
Rare fatalities from hypertension when taken with foods containing tyramine require a restrictive diet that is unpopular with patients. Traditionally used for 'neurotic' or 'atypical' depression. Phenelzine may cause insomnia if taken in the evening.

Other types
Moclobemide
A reversible selective inhibitor of monoamine oxidase A. Its efficacy is similar to most other antidepressants except, perhaps, in severe depression. An alternative for patients not responding to other agents. Side effect profile is relatively benign, and it is generally not necessary to impose a low tyramine diet. Drug interactions may occur. It seems safe in overdoses of up to 20 g.
Nefazodone
A mixed selective serotonin reuptake inhibitor and $5HT_2$ receptor antagonist. Relatively free of gastrointestinal side effects and the sexual dysfunction seen with selective serotonin reuptake inhibitors. More sedative so helps sleep, but some postural hypotension.
Venlafaxine
The first mixed serotonin and noradrenaline reuptake inhibitor (SNRI), with benefits of tricyclic antidepressants and fewer drawbacks. Side effects are nausea, headache and sweating. Anticholinergic and cardiovascular adverse events uncommon, but pre-treatment ECG recommended. It seems safe in overdoses up to 6·75 g. May cause swings into hypomania in patients with bipolar disorders. Rapid onset of action has been observed.

Guidelines on the rational prescribing of antidepressants balance their side effect profile, and hence tolerability and adherence, against cost. Economic studies have tended to show little overall difference in costs between drugs, but costs are distributed between many different budgets and it is often difficult for those paying the immediate purchase cost of a drug to take a global view about savings accruing to others' budgets. Clinically, the choice between antidepressants lies in their safety and tolerability to the patient.

Virtually all available antidepressants are equally effective if given at an adequate dose for a sufficient period

Maintenance treatment

Half of all depressed patients only ever have one episode. The risk of a subsequent episode increases with the number already experienced and with increasing age of onset. As risk of recurrence increases, so prophylactic maintenance treatment should be considered, although most patients hate this. There is good evidence of the efficacy of tricyclic antidepressants for up to five years, but few studies of newer drugs extend beyond one to two years. For long-term treatment, the burden of side effects with the older drugs is a major consideration in choice of treatment.

Non-adherence with antidepressants may reach 50%

Dysthymia

The concept of persistent low-grade depression has changed from a personality disorder to chronic affective disorder (Box 8.6). Hence, past treatment with anxiolytics has now changed to that used in other forms of depression, and there is evidence that most types of antidepressant are effective. However, dysthymic patients may be more sensitive to the side effects of TCAs than those with more severe depression, and, hence, newer antidepressants may be the treatment of choice. The chronic nature of dysthymia may require long-term treatment, particularly when it is associated with episodes of more severe depression (double depression) as recurrence of severe episodes is more likely if the dysthymia is not controlled.

Box 8.6 **Classification of depression***

Primary
Unipolar
- Mixed anxiety and depressive disorder: with prominent anxiety
- Depressive episode: single episode
- Recurrent depressive disorder: recurrent episodes
- Dysthymia: persistent and mild ('depressive personality')
Bipolar
- Bipolar affective disorder: with manic episodes ('manic depression')
- Cyclothymia: persistent instability of mood
Other primary
- Seasonal affective disorder
- Brief recurrent depression

Secondary
May be secondary to medical condition or alcohol or other drugs

Depressive episode
Each episode may be
- Moderate or severe
- With or without somatic syndrome
- If severe, with or without psychotic symptoms

*ICD-10 (*International Classification of Diseases*, 10th edition)

Focused psychotherapies such as cognitive behavioural therapy and marital and family therapies benefit social functioning but have less effect on symptoms. The marked social and interpersonal debility associated with dysthymia and patients' needs to acquire coping skills in managing symptoms and problems suggest that an approach combining antidepressants and focused psychotherapy is most likely to produce lasting benefit.

Psychotic depression

Patients with psychotic depression are the most severely depressed, and they respond poorly to antidepressants alone. Two treatments are effective: combined use of antidepressant and antipsychotic drugs, and electroconvulsive therapy (Box 8.7).

Combining some of the newer antidepressants, particularly the SSRIs, with antipsychotics should be done with caution as inhibition of the liver cytochrome enzymes can raise the plasma concentrations of both drugs, so monitoring may be needed.

Electroconvulsive therapy is an older treatment than antidepressant drugs. It is almost exclusively a hospital-based treatment, and most patients remain as inpatients during the course of treatment. It is particularly effective for severely depressed patients who are either deluded or have marked psychomotor retardation. Treatment entails administering an electric charge to the head of a patient under a general anaesthetic in order to produce a generalised fit. Memory impairment may be reduced by unilateral compared to bilateral administration. From the patients' point of view, they will have a general anaesthetic twice weekly for three to four weeks and experience a mild transient confusional state for an hour or so after each treatment.

Box 8.7 **Electroconvulsive therapy in treating depression**

- The greater the number of typical features of depression, the greater likelihood of a good response to electroconvulsive therapy
- Electroconvulsive therapy is particularly effective in treating depression with psychotic features
- Patients who do not respond to antidepressant drugs may respond to electroconvulsive therapy
- It is essential to continue drug treatment with antidepressants after a successful course of electroconvulsive therapy

Safety of electroconvulsive therapy
- There are no absolute contraindications to its use. Relative contraindications include uncontrolled hypertension, recent myocardial infarction or haemorrhagic stroke
- It may be a life-saving treatment in cases of severe depression
- There is limited evidence that it causes brain damage or permanent intellectual impairment; this must be weighed against its established efficacy in life-threatening severe depression
- Risk of death is similar to that of general anaesthesia for minor surgical procedures – about two deaths per 100,000 treatments
- Several drugs, including selective serotonin reuptake inhibitors, may prolong the duration of the induced seizure

---

Depression and childbearing

Depressive disorders are common in women of childbearing age, and postpartum depression is a serious complication of childbearing. The possibility of pregnancy should be considered in any pre-menopausal woman for whom antidepressant treatment is contemplated. As many pregnancies are unplanned and unintended, contraceptive advice should be given at the outset of treatment and reviewed often, and an antidepressant with little evidence of teratogenicity should be chosen. Where pregnancy is planned, the risks of depression should be weighed against those of ceasing treatment: if antidepressant medication is to be continued, fluoxetine (a SSRI) or possibly imipramine (a TCA) are preferred.

If an unplanned pregnancy occurs while the patient is taking an antidepressant, greatest risk of harm to the foetus occurs in the first 60 days post-conception. During this period, the drug should be stopped or the dose should be reduced as far as practicable. After 60 days, antidepressant treatment may be restarted if thought necessary.

Women with a history of depressive disorders may be at greater risk of developing postnatal depression. Maternal depression has been linked to impaired cognitive and social development in the child. There is little evidence that antidepressants taken during pregnancy provide effective prophylaxis. Treatment involves a combination of antidepressant medication, psychological therapy (there is evidence for CBT), and social support (often involving local organisations for mothers and their children).

Seasonal affective disorder

Symptoms of seasonal affective disorder include typical (low mood and energy) and atypical (increased appetite and sleep) depressive features occurring together in a seasonal pattern. Estimates of prevalence of the disorder in the UK average about 2.5% of the population. A mechanism for the seasonal variation in mood may involve effects of light levels on melatonin metabolism.

Treatment

There is evidence of benefit from phototherapy, although the most effective form of light (short periods of bright light, or gradually increasing intensity mimicking sunrise) is not clear. Patients whose symptoms most closely resemble those typical of depression may respond well to antidepressant medication. Also, antidepressants may have a prophylactic role if started before the typical onset of symptoms in autumn. The value of psychological therapies is unclear.

Bipolar affective disorder

The clinical features of the depressive phase of this illness are identical to those of other depressions, but treatment with antidepressants alone risks drug-induced swings into mania. Effective long-term prophylaxis may be achieved with lithium (this requires pre-treatment screening of renal and thyroid function), sodium valproate or carbamazepine; these treatments are usually initiated by psychiatrists. Bipolar affective disorder is dealt with in Chapter 9.

Suicide and deliberate self-harm

There are about 5000 suicides each year in England and Wales, of which 400–500 involve overdoses of antidepressants. Deliberate self-harm is 20–30 times more common. Not all people who commit suicide have psychiatric illness but, among those who do, depression is the commonest illness and 15% of depressed patients eventually kill themselves.

Assessment of risk is, thus, important and guides treatment (Box 8.8). Many older antidepressants may be fatal in overdose, while the newer effective drugs – such as SSRIs, lofepramine and others – are safer and should be used with high-risk patients. Prescribing should be cautious, for short periods with frequent reviews.

Box 8.8 **Suicide or deliberate self-harm**

Features to be assessed
- Motive
- Circumstances of attempt
- Psychiatric disorder
- Precipitating and maintaining problems
- Coping skills and support
- Risk

High-risk indicators for suicide
- Male
- Age > 40 years
- Family history of suicide
- Unemployed
- Socially isolated
- Suicide note
- Continued desire to die
- Hopelessness, sees no future
- Misuse of drugs or alcohol
- Psychiatric illness (especially depression, but also schizophrenia, personality disorder)

Further information

Bereavement. From: Help the Aged, St James's Walk, London, EC1R 0BE (tel. 0207 278 1114)

Depression and your sex life. From: The Depression Alliance, 35 Westminster Bridge Road, London, SE1 7JB

Down on the farm? Coping with depression in rural areas; a farmer's guide. Available by calling Health Literature Helpline (tel. 0800 555 777)

The experience of grief. From: National Association of Bereavement Services, 4 Pinchin Street, London, E1 6DB (tel. 0207 709 9090)

Personal accounts of mental health problems

Ažman R. *Depra: Living with depression.* Chipmunkapublishing, Brentwood, Essex, 2007. www.chipmunka.com

White C. *Diamonds from coal.* Chipmunkapublishing, Brentwood, Essex, 2005. www.chipmunka.com

Willmott D. *Happy daft.* Chipmunkapublishing, Brentwood, Essex, 2006. www.chipmunka.com

Further reading

Kroenke K, Spitzer RL. The PHQ-9: a new depression diagnostic and severity measure. *Psych Ann* 2002; 32: 509–21.

Mathers CD, Loncar D. Projections of global mortality and burden of disease from 2002 to 2030. *PLoS Med* 2006; 3: e442. doi:10. 1371/journal.pmed.0030442

National Institute for Health and Clinical Excellence. *Depression (amended): Management of depression in primary and secondary care.* NICE guideline CG23. NICE, London, 2007. http://guidance.nice.org.uk/CG23/

The ECT handbook. Council report CR39. Royal College of Psychiatrists, London, 1995.

CHAPTER 9

Bipolar Disorders

Teifion Davies

OVERVIEW

- Several clinical subtypes of the bipolar disorders are recognised: all are life-long, and characterised by periods of disproportionately elevated mood
- Management should focus on the longer term, and aim for maintenance on a single mood stabiliser, although more complex regimens might be required
- Treating depressive phases with an antidepressant alone risks switching to mania
- Insomnia is a critical factor in incipient relapse, and its early management is crucial
- Patients should receive psychological intervention to engage them in active self-management of their disorder

---

Box 9.1 **Clinical subtypes of bipolar mood disorders**

- Mania: episode of elated and excited mood often with psychotic features
- Hypomania: excessive cheerfulness and energy without psychosis
- Bipolar I disorder: recurrent episodes of mania with much less frequent depressive phases
- Bipolar II disorder: recurrent episodes of depression with less frequent hypomanic phases
- Bipolar III disorder: manic episodes triggered by antidepressant treatment of an apparently unipolar depression (also termed switching)
- Rapid cycling bipolar disorder: four or more severe mood episodes occurring in a single year
- Mixed affective state: simultaneous occurrence of features of mania and depression
- Schizoaffective disorder: clear mood (often mania) and schizophrenic features present simultaneously
- Cyclothymia: periodic alternation of mild elation and mild depression (cf. dysthymia)

Bipolar disorders are so-called because, during their course, a patient may experience mood states at either extreme of the mood spectrum. The defining feature of these disorders is abnormal elevation of mood, which is out of proportion to normal happiness. This elation may be accompanied by excessive optimism, impatience, irritability and impaired functioning when it is termed hypomania, or by excitation, excessive activity and often grandiose delusions, that constitute mania. Distinct episodes of depression may also occur, either sequentially or separated by variable periods of normal mood.

Bipolar affective disorder is a life-long, relapsing and remitting illness, with a strong genetic component (almost 70% concordance between monozygotic twins) that affects men and women equally. Its onset is typically in late adolescence or early adult life, and its overall prevalence is about 2% in the population. Clinical subtypes are recognised, with Type I (classical manic-depressive) disorder being slightly less common than Type II (depressive-hypomanic) disorder (Box 9.1). The latter appears to have a younger onset and to be more likely to affect women.

Women with bipolar affective disorder have a high risk of suffering puerperal psychosis in the first three to four weeks following childbirth. An episode of mania follows up to 50% of deliveries to sufferers, compared to one in 500 for women without the disorder.

Diagnosis

Recognition of a typical manic episode is fairly straightforward (Box 9.2). The patient, who may have no previous history of mood disorder, presents with a significant change in mood, activity and thought, which, although it might have been triggered by an identifiable life event, is clearly excessive and disproportionate. Changes may occur abruptly or escalate over a few days. Normal patterns of daily living (notably sleep and appetite) are disrupted, and behaviour is disinhibited, excited, uncontrollable and potentially risky. A rapid flow of grandiose ideas gives rise to pressured and uninterruptible speech. Attempts to calm or contain the patient may be perceived as hostile, and the patient may react with uncharacteristic aggression. Delusions, disordered thought and unintelligible speech may be confused with schizophrenia, while excited and irritable mood may resemble the intense distress and agitation following a major traumatic event.

Hypomania lies on the continuum from normal happiness to abnormal elation, and its diagnosis is less clear-cut. This state lacks psychotic features or significant social impairment, and many patients welcome its increased energy, creativity and sense of well-being. Its presence should alert the doctor to the possibility

ABC of Mental Health, 2nd edition. Edited by T. Davies and T. Craig.
© 2009 Blackwell Publishing, ISBN: 978-0-7279-1639-6.

Mania
- Onset: may be precipitated by life event of personal significance (e.g. bereavement, migration), disrupted circadian rhythms (especially sleep), illness (e.g. endocrinopathy) or childbirth
- Duration: minimum one week for diagnosis; median four months if untreated
- Mood: sustained, inappropriate elation; excessive optimism; constant excitement
- Behaviour: energetic, overactive; socially and sexually disinhibited; excessive spending or dangerous risk-taking; leading to physical exhaustion
- Speech: continuous, pressured, uninterruptible
- Thought: rapidly changing ideas; grandiose delusions (wild schemes, beliefs of personal wealth, status and invulnerability)
- Perception: hallucinations in any modality, often fleeting or rapidly changing
- Biological rhythms: insomnia, lack of appetite and thirst
- Social functioning: disrupted or abandoned

Hypomania
- Onset: precipitating factors may be unclear
- Duration: several days for diagnosis; course may be very variable
- Mood: persistent mild elevation, impatience or irritability
- Behaviour: sociable, inept and inappropriate
- Speech: talkative
- Thought: 'creative', sense of well-being and purpose; no delusions
- Perception: heightened awareness; no hallucinations
- Biological rhythms: impaired but not completely disrupted
- Social functioning: impaired but not completely disrupted

of bipolar II disorder (depression with hypomania) or 'switching' (onset of mania due to treatment of depression).

The depressive phase tends to develop more slowly, although rapid onset of a subjective sense of depression is a common complaint of patients being treated for mania, and may occur while other manic symptoms (especially excess energy) persist. In most respects, the depressive phase resembles a typical episode of unipolar depression and diagnosis depends on similar criteria (see Chapter 8). Untreated depressive episodes have a median duration of six months. Recent studies have found subclinical depression (i.e. persistent depressive symptoms insufficient for diagnosis of a depressive episode) to be present for up to 50% of the time between major episodes. Risk of suicide is greater in bipolar than unipolar depression.

Mixed affective states are particularly unpleasant for the patient, and pose diagnostic difficulties. They are more prolonged than switching or the transition from one mood state to another: features of both mania and depression must coexist for at least two weeks for formal diagnosis. They may be misdiagnosed as personality disorder, especially the emotionally unstable type in which 'mood swings' from day to day occur repetitively from early adolescence. In schizoaffective disorder, clear schizophrenic and affective (usually manic) features are present simultaneously.

Management

Management of bipolar affective disorder is potentially complex (Box 9.3). It must take full account of the medical (diagnosis of bipolar subtype, comorbid conditions), psychological (cognitive patterns, coping strategies) and social (impact on lifestyle and relationships) aspects and their interactions.

Acute management

Acute mania is a medical emergency and may require compulsory admission. Any antidepressant the patient is taking should be stopped. First-line treatment uses antimanic antipsychotic drugs (olanzapine, quetiapine or risperidone) for their tranquillising and antipsychotic effects, and rapid onset of action. Lithium is also effective but its action is delayed until a plasma concentration of about 1 mmol/L is achieved. Valproate is an alternative and may be used to augment an antipsychotic. Sedation with a benzodiazepine (lorazepam or clonazepam) might be necessary. Electroconvulsive therapy has a place in management of severe and intractable mania.

Treatment of acute bipolar depression (a depressive episode in the course of established bipolar disorder) can be particularly problematic. Antidepressants (especially tricyclics) used alone risk switching to mania, rapid cycling or mood destabilisation and 'symptom chasing' in which symptomatic treatment (antidepressants, antipsychotics, sedatives) is given in a vain attempt to achieve control. Ideally, a SSRI should be used in combination with a mood stabilising drug. Quetiapine may be added if an antipsychotic is needed.

If the patient is not under the care of secondary mental health services, referral should be considered whenever additional factors complicate the presentation (Box 9.4). For instance, if the

Box 9.3 **Complexity in managing bipolar disorders**

Biomedical
- Bipolar disorder and its subtypes
- Comorbidity with other disorders

Psychological
- Patterns of thinking and behaviour
- Cognitive impairment

Social
- Lifestyle
- Social impairment

Interaction of all of these

Box 9.4 **Referral to specialist mental health services**

- First episode of mania (including switching from depressive episode)
- Bipolar depression
- Mixed affective state
- Rapid cycling
- Diagnostic difficulty (personality disorder, schizophrenia)
- Comorbidity (anxiety disorders are common; personality disorder; alcohol or illicit drug misuse; physical illness such as renal, thyroid, endocrinopathy)
- Pregnancy or planning family
- Treatment failure
- Risk assessment (risky behaviours, suicide risk)
- Psychosis

Box 9.5 **Principles of managing bipolar disorders**

Strategic
- Long-term perspective
- Broad approach (biological, psychological and social)
- Continuity of care
- Self-management
- Collaboration and concordance

Tactical
- Monitoring
- Recognition
- Early intervention
- Symptom control

Box 9.6 **Practical aspects of managing bipolar disorders**

Do
- Treat disorder not episode: short-term treatment destabilises
- Aim to maintain on single mood stabiliser
- Use symptomatic treatment early (hypnotic or antipsychotic)
- Use antidepressant (SSRI) only with mood stabiliser
- Encourage self-management, especially sleep schedule, drugs, alcohol

Don't
- Don't 'discharge': patients benefit from long-term continuity of care
- Don't prolong symptomatic treatments: taper off rapidly when symptoms controlled
- Don't use tricyclic antidepressants (TCAs): risk of 'switching'
- Don't alter successful regimens: even if idiosyncratic

pattern of the disorder changes (to mixed state or rapid cycling), if monotherapy with an antimanic or mood stabiliser fails or is compromised by comorbid illness, or if the patient's lifestyle changes (pregnancy, risk-taking, substance misuse).

Maintenance

The life-long nature of the disorder means that the principles of chronic disease management apply (Box 9.5). A patient should be engaged actively in the collaborative management of his or her disorder. Treatment should aim to achieve long-term remission, and be designed to accommodate predictable changes in the patient's life. Continuity is crucial, and a patient should have ready access to the same clinician (especially GP) or small team in the long term. The devastating effects of manic episodes justify regular monitoring by a doctor familiar with the patient's relapse pattern, to provide rapid recognition of symptoms, to facilitate early intervention and to control symptoms that would otherwise have produced relapse.

Mood stabilisers

Important decisions include: whether to use a mood stabiliser? If so, which drug? When to start treatment? And, for how long to continue?

Traditionally, mood stabilisers were not used until after a diagnosis of bipolar disorder was established following a second manic episode. As mood stabilising drugs are effective in preventing relapse of mania in 60–70% of cases, their early use is indicated. This is often unacceptable to a young patient following a first episode, so lifestyle advice, and encouragement to seek treatment urgently if symptoms return, might have to suffice (Box 9.6).

Details of starting and monitoring mood stabilisers are given in Chapter 22. Lithium, sodium valproate and olanzapine are all effective in reducing risk of relapse in classical bipolar I disorder. Sodium valproate may also be effective in rapid cycling and mixed states, especially when combined with another mood stabiliser. Carbamazepine is licensed in the UK for use in rapid cycling disorder, but it has complex interactions with other drugs. There is little evidence of efficacy for the other antiseizure agents (except lamotrigine, below).

Mood stabilisers are somewhat less effective in preventing bipolar depression than mania: a 25% reduction in risk of relapse by lithium being the most successful. Antidepressants are used as maintenance treatment after an episode of unipolar depression, but their use in bipolar disorder carries a high risk of switching to mania. Both quetiapine and the antiseizure drug lamotrigine have some efficacy in treating acute depression and reducing the risk of depressive relapse. Inevitably, when no drug stands out, monotherapy must give way to combinations of mood stabiliser and antidepressant; more complex regimens might be needed to treat the protracted depression of bipolar II disorder. Cognitive behavioural therapy (CBT) focusing on depressive cognitions should be combined with medical treatment, and may be as helpful as any single drug.

Many patients find the burden of life-long prophylactic medication intolerable. For those with few previous episodes, stable lifestyles and minimal comorbidity, maintenance medication may be withdrawn cautiously after two to three years free of relapse. For others with more complex histories, more severe episodes, more rapid onset or less stable lifestyle, maintenance treatment should be continued for a longer period, at least five years. For the most severely affected individuals, it may be necessary to continue treatment indefinitely to avoid relapse. Risk of relapse is increased for a period after withdrawal from mood stabilisers, especially lithium: patients should be monitored carefully for at least a year, and warned of the need to seek urgent advice if symptoms recur.

Relapse prevention

Relapse prevention goes beyond medical maintenance treatment to engage the patient in active self-management. A healthy lifestyle including regular exercise, maintenance of social routines and attention to sleep hygiene, are important preventative factors (Box 9.7).

The subjective experiences and overt behaviours that precede a full-blown relapse are highly individual, but their recognition is key to self-management. With the help of carers and family (and ideally friends), the patient should draw up a list of trigger events and activities, and of the resulting marker symptoms of incipient relapse. The list should evolve over time to become increasingly specific for the most significant factors.

Box 9.7 **Key features of a relapse prevention strategy**

Triggers: causes of relapse
- Events, experiences or activities known to precede onset of symptoms
- Disruption of sleep–activity cycle (partying, shift work, jet lag, travel across time zones)
- Excessive use of alcohol or recreational drugs
- Forgeting or rejecting medication

Markers: signs of relapse (only one need be present)
- Agitation, irritability, impatience
- Reduced need for sleep
- Unexplained energy
- Talkative, flirtatious
- Feels 'part of the big picture'

Self-management: participation in control of disorder
- Active control of triggers
- Self-monitoring for markers of relapse
- Cognitive behavioural therapy for depressive features
- Cognitive strategies to cope with life events
- Support from voluntary organisations, and self-help books

Contingency plan: what to do when prevention fails
- A plan constructed with and known to family, friends and doctors
- Includes a supply, and instructions for use, of hypnotic and antipsychotic medication
- Details of key contacts (GP, mental health services)

Psycho-education about the disorder and its management has an important role in facilitating the patient to develop a contingency plan for self-management. This may be combined with CBT to identify his or her dysfunctional behaviour patterns (triggers), recognise early mood changes (markers) and adopt strategies to minimise their effects. Several voluntary organisations and self-help books are available to guide the patient.

Disruption of sleep has a central role in relapse, both as a primary precipitant (e.g. in shift work or jet lag) and as a mediator of other factors such as pain or worry. Insomnia may be the first warning sign of relapse. Patients should be encouraged to hold a contingency supply of a hypnotic or antipsychotic to be taken to prevent a second night of sleep disturbance. This is important as relapse might occur before the patient can gain a consultation with the GP.

Further information

Bipolar Aware, http://www.bipolaraware.co.uk/
- Information
- Self help
Equilibrium – the Bipolar Foundation, http://www.bipolar-foundation.org/
- Information
MDF – the Bipolar Organisation, http://mdf.org.uk/
- Publications and leaflets
- Self-help groups
- Self management training

Personal accounts of mental health problems

Jamison KR. *An unquiet mind: A memoir of moods and madness.* Vintage, New York, 1996.

Pegler J. *A can of madness.* Chipmunkapublishing, Brentwood, Essex, 2002. www.chipmunka.com

Further reading

Department of Health. *The expert patient: A new approach to chronic disease management for the 21st century.* DH, London, 2001.

Hirschfeld RMA: *Guideline watch: Practice guideline for the treatment of patients with bipolar disorder.* American Psychiatric Association, Arlington, VA, 2005. http://www.psych.org/psych_pract/treatg/pg/prac_guide.cfm

Jones S, Haywood P, Lam D. *Coping with bipolar disorder: A guide to living with manic depression.* Oneworld Publications, Oxford, 2002.

National Institute for Health and Clinical Excellence. *Bipolar disorder: The management of bipolar disorder in adults, children and adolescents, in primary and secondary care.* NICE guideline CG38. NICE, London, 2006. http://guidance.nice.org.uk/CG38/

Perry A, Tarrier N, Morriss R, *et al.* Randomised controlled trial of efficacy of teaching patients with bipolar disorder to identify early symptoms of relapse and obtain treatment. *BMJ* 1999; **318**: 149–53.

Scott AIF (ed.). *The ECT Handbook*, 2nd edn. Council Report CR128. Royal College of Psychiatrists, London, 2005.

Tondo L. Bipolar disorder. In: Griez EJL, Faravelli C, Nutt DJ, Zohar J, eds. *Mood disorders: Clinical management and research issues.* John Wiley, Chichester, 2005: 103–16.

Young AH, Hammond JM. Lithium in mood disorders: increasing evidence base, declining use? *Br J Psych* 2007; **191**: 474–6.

CHAPTER 10

Schizophrenia

Trevor Turner

OVERVIEW

- Schizophrenia is a relatively common, severe and enduring psychotic disorder of multifactorial aetiology, with a variety of presentations

- There is an increased relative risk of suicide and of premature death linked to lifestyle and physical ill health; but violence is relatively rare

- Antipsychotic drug treatment is central to management, but psychological and social approaches are important at varying stages of the illness

- Early recognition and treatment with antipsychotic drugs will minimise long-term social impairment; about 70% of patients remain symptom-free with long-term treatment and social support

Schizophrenia is a relatively common form of psychotic disorder (severe mental illness). Its lifetime prevalence is nearly 1%, its annual incidence is about 10–15 per 100,000, and in the UK the average general practitioner cares for 10–20 schizophrenic patients depending on the location and social surroundings of the practice. Symptoms are termed 'positive' or 'negative', depending on whether they are psychological add-ons (e.g. delusions) or deficits (e.g. anhedonia) such that it is a syndrome with various presentations and a variable, often relapsing, long-term course.

Although schizophrenia is publicly misconceived as 'split personality', the diagnosis has good reliability, even across ages and cultures, though there is no biochemical marker. Onset before the age of 30 is the norm, with men tending to present some four years younger than women. Clues as to aetiology are tantalising, and management remains endearingly clinical.

Aetiology

Evidence for a genetic cause grows stronger: up to 50% of identical (monozygotic) twins will share a diagnosis, compared with about 15% of non-identical (dizygotic) twins. The strength of genetic factors varies across families, but some 10% of a patient's first-degree relatives (parents, siblings and children) will also be schizophrenic as will 50% of the children of two schizophrenic parents.

Pre-morbid abnormalities of speech and behaviour may be present during childhood. The role of obstetric complications and viral infection *in utero* remains unproved. Enlarged ventricles and abnormalities of the temporal lobes are not uncommon findings from neuroimaging. Thus, a picture is emerging of a genetic condition, enhanced or brought out by subtle forms of environmental damage: a neurodevelopmental disorder. The possible role of psycho-active agents such as cannabis is much debated (use in early teenage being associated with later schizophrenia), whereas season of birth, immigration and urbanisation also seem contributory.

> Symptoms are characterised most usefully as positive or negative, although the traditional diagnostic subcategories (hebephrenic, paranoid, catatonic and simple) have mixtures of both

Clinical features

Positive symptoms and signs

These are essentially disordered versions of the normal brain functions of thinking, perceiving, formation of ideas and sense of self (Box 10.1). Patients with thought disorder may present with complaints of poor concentration or of their mind being blocked or emptied (thought block): a patient stopping in a perplexed fashion while in mid-speech and the interviewer having difficulty in following the speech are typical signs.

Hallucinations

These are false perceptions in any of the senses in the absence of real external stimuli: a patient experiences a seemingly real voice or smell, for example, although nothing actually occurred. The hallmark of schizophrenia is that patients experience voices talking about them as 'he' or 'she' (third person auditory hallucinations), but second person 'command' voices also occur, as do olfactory, tactile (both somatic and visceral) and visual hallucinations. Functional MRI research indicates that misattribution of self-generated 'inner' perceptions may account for such experiences.

ABC of Mental Health, 2nd edition. Edited by T. Davies and T. Craig.
© 2009 Blackwell Publishing, ISBN: 978-0-7279-1639-6.

Delusions

These are abnormal beliefs held with absolute certainty, dominating the patient's mind, and untenable in terms of the sociocultural background. Delusions often derive from attempts to make sense of other symptoms such as the experience of passivity (sensing that someone or something is controlling one's body, emotions or thoughts). Typical experiences are of thoughts being taken or sucked out of the head (a patient insisted that her mother was 'stealing her brain') or inserted into the mind, or of one's thoughts being known to others (respectively termed thought withdrawal, thought insertion and thought broadcast). Cult beliefs in telepathy and mind control may relate to partial forms of these experiences.

Negative symptoms

A negative symptom is the absence of some ability or attribute a normal person would possess. These include loss of personal abilities such as initiative, interest in others and the sense of enjoyment (anhedonia). Blunted or fatuous emotions (flat affect), limited speech and much time spent doing nothing are typical behaviours. Subtle cognitive deficits often persist (or even worsen) despite continuing treatment.

Forms of schizophrenia

Paranoid schizophrenia, the most common form, is dominated by florid, positive symptoms, especially delusions, that may build into a complex conspiracy theory that seems initially quite credible. The term paranoid has a broader meaning than persecutory, defining a sense of things around one having special, personal significance. Thus, car lights flashing may be evidence that the IRA are following you or proof that a film star is in love with you. The more bizarre the beliefs, the easier the diagnosis.

In contrast, those presenting only with negative symptoms are described as having simple schizophrenia, whereas hebephrenia is a mix of negative and positive symptoms with insidious onset in adolescence.

The early stages of schizophrenic illnesses can vary considerably. A typical presentation is a family's concerns that a personality has changed or an insistence that a son 'must be on drugs'. A decline in personal hygiene, loss of jobs and friends for no clear reason, and depressive symptoms mixed with a degree of ill-defined perplexity are all common. About one in 10 commit suicide, usually as younger patients. It is relatively rare for sufferers to assault others although criminality rates are increased. There is an increased relative risk of premature death, linked to lifestyle and physical ill health.

Diagnosis remains a clinical skill requiring a good social history corroborated by others as well as a detailed assessment of the patient's mental state

Diagnosis

Presentations evolve over time, from non-specific depression or anxiety into overt psychotic states with typical symptoms. Differential diagnosis is limited, but routine blood tests, a urine screen for drug metabolites and special investigations are useful to exclude rarer conditions. Complex partial seizures (temporal lobe epilepsy), cerebral lesions, hypothyroidism (in older patients) and systemic lupus erythematosus are possibilities. The hallucinations associated with alcoholism, illicit drugs and medications should also be considered, although some 50% of schizophrenic patients show comorbid drug abuse.

Management

Management requires pharmacological, psychological and social approaches, depending on the stage of the illness.

Drug treatment

Early treatment with antipsychotic drugs, minimising the 'duration of untreated psychosis' (DUP) is central to resolving unpleasant symptoms and social impairment (Box 10.2). National Institute for Health and Clinical Excellence guidelines recommend 'atypical' antipsychotics as first-line treatment (i.e. olanzapine, risperidone and quetiapine), although they are probably no more effective than the traditional dopamine blockers (e.g. haloperidol, chlorpromazine). Only risperidone is available as a depot preparation, and they vary in their sedating properties, weight gain and hyperglycaemia.

Continuing treatment

Depot injections giving slow, stable release of drugs over one to four weeks are extremely useful. They enhance compliance, a particular problem in those patients who lack insight. Relief of symptoms is achieved in at least 70% of patients who are maintained on regular medication of whatever type. Some 30–40% of patients with treatment-resistant illnesses respond to some degree to atypical clozapine, which requires regular haematological testing because of a 1–2% agranulocytosis rate.

Side effects are a particular problem, especially with dopamine blockers. Parkinsonian symptoms require antimuscarinic drugs (such as procyclidine or orphenadrine) in a third or more of patients. Sedation or a sense of feeling flattened or depressed may also be distressing. Restlessness, either psychological or affecting the legs (akathisia), is poorly understood but can respond to β-blockers. Benzodiazepines usefully treat common problems such as excessive arousal or anxiety or difficulties in sleeping.

The 'atypical' antipsychotic drugs, such as clozapine or risperidone, have an additional blocking action on serotonin receptors that seems to reduce side effects and negative symptoms. Development of such 'cleaner' drugs is one of the most exciting aspects of research in managing schizophrenia. Aripiprazole appears to cause fewer metabolic side effects, and quetiapine less hyperprolactinaemia, than other atypical drugs (Box 10.3).

Psychological treatment

Psychological interventions are based on cognitive behavioural therapy (CBT), which for many patients can reduce the impact of hallucinations and delusional beliefs, the use of insight-orientated psycho-education (for patients and carers) and family work (Box 10.4).

Box 10.2 Advantages of early recognition and treatment

Minimises
- Subjective distress
- Positive symptoms
- Anxiety and depression

Reduces
- Frequency of relapse
- Cognitive deterioration
- Loss of personal self-care skills

Limits
- Social disruption and deterioration
- Loss of family support and social networks
- Loss of interpersonal skills

Box 10.3 Side effects of antipsychotic drugs

Immediate
- Acute dystonias and dyskinaesias
- Sedation
- Dry mouth
- Hypotension
- Akathisia
- Constipation
- Oculogyric crisis
- Neuroleptic malignant syndrome

Medium term (weeks)
- Raised prolactin concentrations, leading to:
  - Amenorrhoea
  - Subfertility
  - Impotence
- Prolonged QTc interval and dysrhythmias
- Weight gain and metabolic syndrome

Long term (months)
- Tardive dyskinaesia

Box 10.4 Psychological and social interventions

With patient
- Training in daily living skills
- Training in social skills
- Insight work
- Training in job skills
- Training in anxiety and 'stress' management
- Cognitive therapy for delusions and hallucinations

With patient's family
- Information and support
- Education about illness and its effects
- Telephone helpline for out of hours support
- Self-help and carers groups
- Family therapy to reduce high expressed emotion

Relapse in schizophrenia seems closely associated with the level of the family's emotional expression as measured by formal assessments of critical comments or expressed hostility in family interviews. Fashionable theories of causation in the 1960s, which designated the 'schizophrenogenic' parent, have now been discarded. There is, however, a close association between high arousal in the family and early relapse: this can be lowered by structured family education, reducing face-to-face contact via attendance at a day centre and formal family therapy.

> **Psychological interventions can minimise distress and reduce frequency of relapse**

Social support

Community mental health teams (CMHTs; Chapter 6) are the multidisciplinary backbone for help with medication, disability benefits and housing needs. Hostels or group homes vary in structure and support, from the high dependence units that provide 24-hour care to the semi-independence of a supported flat with someone visiting daily or less often. Day care, whether an active rehabilitation unit aimed at developing job skills or simply support with low key activities, can improve personal functioning (for example hygiene, conversation and friendships) as well as ensuring early detection of relapse.

There is evidence that assertive outreach support may reduce the need for respite admissions and length of admission. However, the myth that community care supplants the need for hospital beds is being superseded, particularly where there are high levels of homelessness, such as in the inner cities. A ratio of one acute bed for 10 community placements is probably acceptable.

> **Social interventions are the cornerstone of community care**

Prognosis

Prognosis depends on presentation, response to treatment, and the quality of aftercare. Early and continued medication remains the key to good management. Acute onset over several weeks rather than many months, a supportive family, personal intelligence and insight, positive rather than negative symptoms, a later age of onset (over 25 years) and a good response to low doses of drugs are indicative of a better outcome. By contrast, the worst case scenario would be an insidious illness over several years in a teenager from a disrupted family who shows possible brain damage or additional learning difficulties (Box 10.5).

What is clear is that the residual population of the old asylums – incontinent, mute and utterly dependent – is largely a thing of the past. However, a younger group of constantly relapsing patients ('revolving-door patients') shows the limitations of community support. Failure to comply with medication is often a key factor, and targeted Early Intervention Services (see Chapter 6) using multidisciplinary approaches to first-onset illnesses are showing some success.

Outlook

The development of local guidelines and supportive general practices or psychiatric liaison clinics are both educational and effective. Stigma and media hype of 'untoward incidents' (e.g. homicides) tend to mask the good stability and personal functioning of the great majority of patients. Human resources in the form of community psychiatric nurses, social workers, occupational therapists and care workers are often underestimated as well as under-funded.

Excellent information is obtainable from voluntary groups such as Rethink or the Hearing Voices Network. New drug and psychological treatments, as well as research insights into the differing syndromes and symptoms, give hope for the future

Schizophrenia remains a diagnostic, clinical and rehabilitative challenge

Mania and other psychoses

Psychotic symptoms, often indistinguishable from those seen in schizophrenia, occur in bipolar affective disorder (manic–depressive illness). Mania typically presents with hyperactivity, an elevated or excessively irritable mood, sleep loss, pressure of speech and a tendency to jump from topic to topic (flight of ideas). The latter may mimic forms of thought disorder, while grandiose beliefs (often delusional) may generate excess spending or a chaotic personal lifestyle. Hypomania is the term applied to a less severe form without psychotic features.

Modern classification systems recognise the existence of acute and transient psychotic disorders, often occurring in association with stress, which may resolve spontaneously in a few days or weeks. On the other hand, persistent delusional disorder is characterised by circumscribed delusional beliefs of long standing in the absence of other psychotic features or of intellectual deterioration. Schizophrenic or manic symptoms may arise in a range of infective disorders (such as malaria and HIV infection), metabolic disorders (such as hypothyroidism) and idiopathic cerebral disorders.

Personal accounts of mental health problems

Geraghty D. *Cracking and barkin'*. Chipmunkapublishing, Brentwood, Essex, 2007. www.chipmunka.com

Sen D. *The world is full of laughter*. Chipmunkapublishing, Brentwood, Essex, 2002. www.chipmunka.com

Further reading

Adams CE, Fenton MK, Quraishi S, David AS. Systematic meta-review of depot anti-psychotic drugs for people with schizophrenia. *Br J Psych* 2001; **179**: 290–9.

Barrowclough C, Tarrier N. *Families of schizophrenic patients: Cognitive behavioural intervention*. Chapman & Hall, London, 1992.

Haro J *et al.* Remission and relapse in the outpatient care of schizophrenia – 3 year result from the Schizophrenia Outpatient Health Outcomes Study (SOHO). *J Clin Psychopharmacol* 2006; **26**: 571–8.

National Institute for Health and Clinical Excellence. *Schizophrenia: Core interventions in the treatment and management of schizophrenia in primary and secondary care*. NICE guideline CG1. NICE, London, 2002. http://guidance.nice.org.uk/CG1/

National Institute for Health and Clinical Excellence. *Bipolar disorder: The management of bipolar disorder in adults, children and adolescents, in primary and secondary care*. NICE guideline CG38. NICE, London, 2006. http://guidance.nice.org.uk/CG38/

Woolley J, McGuire P. Neuroimaging in schizophrenia: what does it tell the clinician? *Adv Psych Treat* 2005; **11**: 195–202.

CHAPTER 11

Disorders of Personality

Martin Marlowe

OVERVIEW

- Personality disorder involves pervasive and inflexible patterns of thinking, feeling and behaving that are evident from childhood and cause distress to the individual and his or her community

- Several subtypes are described but for clinical purposes three 'clusters' are recognised: odd-eccentric, dramatic, histrionic

- Psychological interventions using focused psychodynamic psychotherapy or dialectical behaviour therapy are preferable to drug treatments

- Inpatient treatment is unusual, and should be voluntary, well planned and ideally to a specialist unit

The 200-year history of personality disorder is characterised by a confusion of terminology, derived from different theoretical perspectives but describing a well-recognised group of patients. The diagnosis has been seen as unreliable, perceived as a pejorative label and seen as synonymous with therapeutic nihilism. However, recent research is beginning to provide a more optimistic view of these conditions.

Describing disorders of personality

Personality can be described in terms of 'characteristics' or 'types'. The dimensional approach involves describing the degree to which an individual displays particular characteristics (e.g. impulsivity, novelty-seeking) to generate a profile for that individual. This approach marries well with attempts to describe normal personality variation and with investigation of possible biological associations. However, there is no consensus as to which characteristics best describe disorders of personality and the origins of the term personality disorder lie in the description of psychopathology rather than the study of personality.

The traditional approach to diagnosis requires the presence of specific, distinct features of a type of personality disorder. This categorical approach underpins the major classifications. The World Health Organization's *International Classification of Diseases*, 10th edition (ICD-10) provides descriptions of eight disorders with

diagnostic guidelines and the American Psychiatric Association's *Diagnostic and Statistical Manual*, 4th edition (DSM-IV) provides twelve (Box 11.1). The types are broadly similar but the systems have important differences. For the past 25 years, the latter system has encouraged clinicians to assess individuals along five separate axes with the presence or absence of personality disorder rated on Axis II and major psychiatric disorders along Axis I. This overcomes the false dichotomy of an individual having either a personality disorder or another condition. The former does not confer immunity against the latter and often both coexist.

The DSM-IV also groups similar types of disorder into three clusters: Cluster A includes individuals perceived as odd or eccentric and includes schizotypal personality disorder (which is classified with schizophrenia-like conditions in ICD-10). Cluster B has been referred to as the 'dramatic' cluster with more overt behavioural disturbances being typical. This group includes borderline, histrionic, antisocial and narcissistic disorders. Cluster C brings together disorders of the anxious, dependent and avoidant type.

The term 'psychopathic disorder' is not a clinical diagnosis but was a legal term defined in the Mental Health Act 1983. A new portmanteau term 'dangerous and severe personality disorder' is now in use although its clinical relevance is unclear.

Box 11.1 **Classifications of personality disorder**

WHO (ICD-10)	APA (DSM-IV)
Paranoid	Cluster A
Schizoid	Paranoid
	Schizoid
	Schizotypal
Dissocial	Cluster B
Histrionic	Antisocial
Emotionally unstable (with impulsive and borderline subtypes)	Histrionic
	Borderline
	Narcissistic
Anankastic	Cluster C
Dependent	Obsessive–compulsive
Anxious	Dependent
	Avoidant
	Passive aggressive

ABC of Mental Health, 2nd edition. Edited by T. Davies and T. Craig.
© 2009 Blackwell Publishing, ISBN: 978-0-7279-1639-6.

The ICD-10 recognises a group of habit and impulse disorders including behavioural syndromes such as pathological gambling, fire setting (pyromania), stealing (kleptomania) and hair pulling (trichotillomania). Elaboration of physical symptoms for psychological reasons, and intentional production of symptoms (factitious disorder) are also included (Box 11.2).

Epidemiology

Differences in case-definition may well be a factor in the wide variation in the prevalence of personality disorder in the community, estimates ranging from 4–13% of the general population. What seems clearer is the trend toward higher prevalence in more institutional settings with levels of 40–60% in secondary care, 36–67% in psychiatric inpatients and up to 78% in prison populations. Personality disorder is unlikely to be the presenting problem in primary care but is associated with higher frequency of consultation and use of psychotropic medication, and more difficult help-seeking behaviour (Box 11.3). Disorders in Cluster C may predominate in rural areas, whereas Cluster B disorders predominate in urban settings.

Prevalence tends to be higher in younger age groups and is approximately equal for men and women overall. However, some disorders are diagnosed more often in men (antisocial personality disorder), others in women (borderline and histrionic disorders), and the diagnosis tends to be made more often in UK white than UK black individuals. A diagnosis of personality disorder is associated with long-term unemployment, the experience of more adverse life events, and, in Cluster B, alcohol and illicit substance misuse, deliberate self-harm (60–80%) and completed suicide (approximately 9%).

Aetiology

The notion of personality disorder as an attenuated form of major illness persists with the relation of Cluster A disorders to the schizophrenia spectrum, and Cluster C to a more general anxiety syndrome. Nearly two-thirds of the variation in the population can be attributed to genotypic variation for Clusters C and B and a little over one-third for Cluster A. From a dimensional perspective, it has been argued that key characteristics of novelty-seeking, harm-avoidance and reward-dependence are modulated by dopaminergic, serotonergic and noradrenergic systems, respectively. Separate investigations have linked lowered central serotonin levels with greater impulsivity.

Cluster B disorders remain the most intensively investigated categories with subtle disorders of executive functioning and reduced pre-frontal lobe functioning being associated with antisocial personality disorder and behaviour. Borderline personality disorder has been associated with impaired attention and memory, processing of emotions and decision-making, as well as pre-frontal cortex, cingulate gyrus and amygdala dysfunction. It has been suggested that these individuals also show excessive physiological reactivity to stress as a result of traumatic early life experiences (Box 11.4).

Psychological theories of these disorders relate adverse early life experiences and problems in early attachment to later problems in emotional development and interpersonal relationships. Traditionally, this has formed one part of the nature versus nurture debate. Recent investigations suggest that what we bring to the world (genetically) has a bearing on how we respond to the world (life events in particular) and indeed what we elicit from the world. These gene–environment interactions may play a more powerful role in development, either as protective or vulnerability factors, than genetic or environmental factors in isolation.

Assessment of personality disorder

Patients with personality disorder may present with a range of behavioural, emotional or associated problems (Box 11.5).

Box 11.2 **Common themes in definitions of personality disorder**

Inclusions
- Repetitive behaviours, emotional responses and/or views of self or other
- These are pervasive and inflexible
- Are outside the individual's cultural or subcultural norm
- Evident in early life and persist into adulthood
- Lead to distress or dysfunction in work or relationships or both

Exclusions
- Other psychiatric disorder
- Physical disorder
- Alcohol/substance misuse

Box 11.3 **Reasons for referring to specialist services**

- Diagnostic uncertainty and comorbidity
- Risk assessment and management
- Specialist prescribing
- Admission

Box 11.4 **Enduring personality changes**

Previous personality may change permanently after catastrophic experiences in adult life (such as hostage-taking, torture or other disaster) or severe mental illness

---

Box 11.5 **Common presentations of personality disorder**

- Aggression
- Anxiety and depression
- Bingeing, vomiting, purging and other eating problems
- Alcohol and substance misuse
- Deliberate self-harm

Those with Cluster A problems may be less likely to present, but the distinction to be made will be between personality disorder and psychotic illness. For Cluster B, aggression (toward themselves or others), fluctuating mood, anxiety, depression, problems with eating, alcohol and substance misuse, may be the initial presenting features. In Cluster C disorders, depression and anxiety may predominate.

Assessment involves taking a detailed history with particular attention to early experience, behaviour and events, in addition to the individual's reaction to them and the context in which they occurred. The individual's personal history is continued into adulthood, covering work, relationships, alcohol and substance misuse, forensic history and current social circumstances. The aims are to establish whether there are recurring patterns of behaviour or emotional response and the impact of any emerging patterns on relationships, work and overall level of function.

The individual's psychiatric and medical histories are important in identifying any exclusion to the diagnosis, past interventions and their effects positive or negative. Mental state examination is needed to identify comorbid conditions or exclusions.

> **A patient's current mental state can influence the history given, and so it is very unlikely that a diagnosis of personality disorder can be made at first meeting**

With the patient's consent a collateral history can highlight issues the individual may not appreciate, although the effect of chronic major illness on the carer's perception of the patient needs to be considered also. General practitioners are often in a good position to assess what represents a change in a patient's personality (suggestive of illness) and what is a continuation or exacerbation of pre-existing problems (Box 11.6).

Box 11.6 Prerequisites for diagnosis of personality disorder

Patient displays a pattern of
- behaviour
- perception of self, others and the environment
- emotional response

that is
- evident in early life
- pervasive
- a deviation from patient's cultural norm
- persists into adulthood
- inflexible

and leads to
- distress to self, others or society
- dysfunction in interpersonal, social or working relationships

but is not attributable to
- other psychiatric disorder (such as schizophrenia, depression, drug misuse)
- other physical disorder (such as acute intoxication, organic brain disease)

Interventions

The basic principle in any intervention is the provision of a plan with realistic objectives that is readily understood by all involved. This often proves difficult in practice, and mutual support in delivering a plan of care requires dedicated time and perseverance. Planning for crises can prove more effective than reacting to them as they occur (Box 11.7). The development of a therapeutic relationship with the patient and their engagement in the process of planning care are early goals in addressing the problems. It is likely that someone with difficulties in forming and maintaining relationships will also have problems in relating to those who are trying to help. A clear, consistent approach aids the development of a working relationship.

Psychological interventions

From the relatively limited evidence to date (referring largely to borderline personality disorder), psychological approaches are preferable to drug treatments which are seen largely as adjunctive. Specialist services have been described involving focused psychodynamic psychotherapy following brief inpatient admission (Box 11.8), supported by attendance at a structured day programme. Whilst benefits in mood and reduction in self-harm may not be apparent immediately, the gains appear to be made after the first six months of the intervention (Box 11.9). Dialectical behaviour therapy (DBT) involves a combination of practical support, help in coping with stress without self-harm, emotional support to address early traumatic life experiences and help in changing the 'black and white' polarised views that might have become habitual ways of thinking. Early gains in reduced self-harm have been reported although the effects may wane by 12 months.

Box 11.7 General principles of intervention

- Be realistic about what can be delivered, by whom and in what period
- Avoid being cast as angel or tyrant
- Communicate clearly with the patient and other professionals involved
- Aim for a stable, long-term therapeutic relationship: this can be achieved with a fairly low level of contact
- Aim to improve the patient's
  - self-worth
  - problem-solving abilities in the short run
  - motivation for change in the long run

Box 11.8 Inpatient admission for personality disorder

Ideally admissions should be
- Planned with the patient, the inpatient unit and community team
- For a mutually agreed purpose
- For a mutually agreed brief period
- On a voluntary basis
- With an agreed plan of discharge to specified follow-up

Therapeutic communities are available within and outside NHS provision: they share the aim of enabling the patient to address problems and change behaviour through living in an environment shared with others with broadly similar problems, and participating in groups to share and confront problems as they arise. The emphasis is on community rather than hospital, with residents taking responsibility at all levels of managing each other's difficulties and the environment itself. It appears that better outcome is associated with longer stay, residents expecting to stay for around 12 months. Cognitive analytic and cognitive behavioural therapy have also been reported to be of benefit although the indicators of benefit are less clear. Overall, psychotherapy may well be the preferred intervention but is probably best delivered in the context of a structured care plan (Box 11.10).

Medication

Antidepressants have proved to be of equivocal benefit for depressive symptoms in borderline personality disorder, although there is some support for the use of phenelzine. The side effects and toxicity in overdose may outweigh potential benefits, however. Fluoxetine has been reported to reduce impulsive aggression. There have been concerns over the safety of selective serotonin reuptake inhibitors (SSRIs) and similar issues have been raised for tricyclic antidepressants in borderline patients, although their anxiolytic effects may be of benefit in those with Cluster C disorders.

Box 11.9 Practical points in managing deliberate self-harm

- Admit patients to hospital only as part of a carefully prepared treatment plan
- Treat physical injuries appropriately
- Relative indications for admission are for assessment of coexisting illness or risk of suicide
- Inpatient contracts, drawn up and signed by patient and staff, have been advocated and may provide a patient with the necessary structure within which help can be offered and received
- The content of a contract must be carefully considered if it is to be a constructive tool rather than a prescription of punishment
- When available, specialist inpatient units allow a much better opportunity for changing recurrent self-harm than do general psychiatric units

---

Box 11.10 Core features of psychological interventions in borderline personality disorder

- Structured meetings with consistent approach
- Focused on enabling self-reflection and self-care
- Long-term commitment
- Approach is understandable to the patient
- Supported by additional services and crisis plan
- Therapists are supported themselves

Box 11.11 Prescribing for patients with personality disorder

- Agree target symptom and record it
- Agree simplest medication regimen, and provide written information about drugs
- Agree trial of specific duration
- Prescribe in limited supply with regular review of risks and benefits
- End trial if risk greater than benefit or ineffective
- Avoid polypharmacy
- Avoid benzodiazepines

Other drugs

Mood stabilisers (lithium, carbamazepine and sodium valproate) have been reported to reduce levels of aggression, and to reduce mood fluctuations. Tolerability, toxicity in overdose and adverse risk/benefit considerations limit their use. Traditional antipsychotics have shown some benefits in isolated older studies, e.g. flupenthixol reducing repeated self-harm and haloperidol reducing irritability. Atypical antipsychotics may prove to be better tolerated and there is some limited evidence for the use of quetiapine and clozapine in borderline patients. Olanzapine is currently under investigation in this group.

At the present time, however, the evidence base does not support more than a therapeutic trial of medications in borderline personality disorder. Use for this purpose would be outside UK licences for these drugs and so protocols for prescribing in these circumstances should be consulted (Box 11.11).

Conclusion

Overall, the past 10 years have seen a greater interest in research into disorders of personality and interventions that might help. The next advance will need to be in service development to keep pace with the research findings.

Further reading

American Psychiatric Association. *DSM-IV: Diagnostic and statistical manual of mental disorders*, 4th edn. APA, Washington, DC, 1994.

Bateman AW, Tyrer P. Effective management of personality disorder. http://www.dh.gov.uk/prod_consum_dh/idcplg?IdcService=GET_FILE&dID=23336&Rendition=Web

National Institute for Health and Clinical Excellence. *Self-harm: The short-term physical and psychological management and secondary prevention of self-harm in primary and secondary care*. NICE guideline CG16. NICE, London, 2004. http://guidance.nice.org.uk/CG16/

National Institute for Mental Health in England. *Personality disorder: No longer a diagnosis of exclusion*. Department of Health, London, 2003. http://www.dh.gov.uk/en/Publicationsandstatistics/Publications/PublicationsPolicyAndGuidance/DH_4009546

World Health Organization. *The ICD-10 classification of mental and behavioural disorders. Clinical descriptions and diagnostic guidelines*. WHO, Geneva, 1992.

CHAPTER 12

Psychosexual Problems

Dinesh Bhugra, James P Watson and Teifion Davies

OVERVIEW

- Up to 50% of people experience psychosexual difficulties with sexual dysfunction being the most common problem
- Biological, psychological and environmental or cultural factors may contribute to the disorder and its presentation
- Assessment must take account of the relationship within which sexual activity takes place or is desired: prognosis is poor if only one partner (the identified patient) attends sessions
- Drug treatment may give symptomatic relief from erectile dysfunction but psychological intervention will be required for longer term improvement
- Paraphilias are sexual preferences that the patient or others find unacceptable: they may result in law breaking, and require specialist assessment

Psychosexual problems of different kinds are universal and are prevalent across cultures. The purpose of sex can be seen as a procreative or pleasurable activity and this may influence the pathway the individual takes in seeking help. In assessing and managing psychosexual problems counsellors, sex therapists, urologists, general practitioners and psychiatrists can help. Other medical professionals such as physicians and gynaecologists may be involved. Origins of psychosexual dysfunction may involve complex and multiple aetiological factors. Patterns of communication and marital relationships also play a role. Sexual dysfunction is relatively common and between 26% and 50% of people have reported it in some surveys.

Relationship and sexual problems

Sexual problems must be evaluated in terms of the relationships in which they are manifest. Relationships can be classified as stable or unstable and satisfactory or unsatisfactory, and most relationship problems can be thought of as including difficulties with communication, conflict and commitment. Difficulties tend to vary at different stages of longstanding relationships such as marriage,

ABC of Mental Health, 2nd edition. 2009. Edited by T. Davies and T. Craig. © 2009 Blackwell Publishing, ISBN: 978-0-7279-1639-6.

accompanying the couple's advancing years. Many sexual problems occur because of threatened or actual rupture of a relationship or separation (including death of a partner).

Close relationships are shaped by the experiences and expectations of the couples and by legal and cultural influences. Three areas commonly require evaluation: implications of unmarried cohabitation rather than marriage, different traditions of relationships in different cultural groups (such as whether marriage partners should be arranged by parents or chosen by the young people) and strong religious beliefs.

Sexual problems

Four main classes of sexual problems are encountered in clinical practice: sexual dysfunctions (the most common), sexual drive problems, gender problems, and sexual variations and deviations. About 10% of patients attending general practice have some kind of current sexual or relationship difficulty. Three general points are important:

- People vary greatly in the quantity and type of sexual activity they seek to undertake, and in its importance for them
- Whenever a substantial relationship difficulty accompanies sexual dysfunction, one partner is usually the referred patient, but a joint meeting with both partners should be offered. The prognosis is poor if both do not attend for joint meetings
- While it is often easy to identify specifically sexual aspects of a problem, it is difficult to evaluate a couple's relationship from a brief assessment.

Sexual dysfunctions

These are problems that make sexual intercourse difficult or impossible. They may be primary (intercourse never adequate) or secondary (intercourse adequate at some time in the past). Erectile and ejaculatory difficulties have similar causes and respond to similar treatments in both heterosexual and homosexual couples.

Classification of sexual dysfunction

Basic classification of sexual dysfunction relies on three phases of sexual activity: desire, arousal and orgasm. An additional category is for pain during or after sexual intercourse. In the phases of desire and arousal, increased or decreased activity are easily identifiable; similarly, early or delayed orgasm are clearly identifiable in this phase.

Additional factors that must be taken into account include sexual orientation, age, infertility, religious, educational and social states, and history of child sex abuse. Culture-bound syndromes such as dhat or koro may present as sexual dysfunction (see Chapter 19).

Causes of sexual dysfunction

Efficient sexual function requires anatomical integrity, intact vascular and neurological function, and adequate hormonal control. Peripheral genital efficiency is modulated by excitatory and inhibitory neural connections that mediate psychological influences, which, in turn, are affected by environmental factors.

Sexual dysfunctions are rarely caused by a single factor, although one may predominate. The question is not, 'Is this problem physical or psychological?' but 'How much of each kind of factor operates in this case?' Similar causative factors operate in men and women, but their manifestations are more obvious in men. It is easy to overlook women's problems unless special inquiry is made.

Biological factors occur often in the course of chronic physical and mental illnesses. Hypogonadism is a well-recognised cause, but is not common. Sexual difficulties are rarely due to testosterone deficiency in men or menopausal or menstrual irregularities in women, though the possibility is often entertained, perhaps because doctors are less comfortable evaluating psychological and relationship factors. It is often the case that no definite biological cause can be found in a particular patient, and other mechanisms are presumed to operate.

Selective serotonin reuptake inhibitors (SSRIs) are well known to cause sexual dysfunction, especially paroxetine, fluoxetine and sertraline. Tricyclic antidepressants can cause differential effects on domains of sexual functioning. Moclobemide and bupropion are said to have less sexual side effects. Antipsychotics such as thioridazine produce various sexual side effects, although the data are mixed. Even atypical antipsychotics such as olanzapine and clozapine cause sexual dysfunction. In managing sexual dysfunction under these circumstances dose reduction, drug holidays and adjuvant therapies may help.

During development, individuals acquire from their experiences of care givers and other personal models a concept of what people are like. Traumatic experiences with adults during childhood may contribute to later sexual and relationship preferences. However, there is no specific connection between particular experiences of early abuse and later problems, and it is remarkable how often people with awful early experiences emerge relatively intact. Nevertheless, the responses of an adult to a prospective sexual partner are framed by expectations of how 'a person like that' will behave.

Cognitions (thoughts) and moods (emotions) shape each person's experience of sexual arousal and behaviour. Attentional processes are important: in the common experience of spectatoring, people focus on their own performance, often expecting failure, rather than on the sensuality of lovemaking. Pain, ruminations and worries divert attention.

Intense negative emotions tend to reduce sexual activity and performance, but the association is not close. In depression, sexual enjoyment is often diminished but occasionally increased; the preferred erotic behaviour may alter, often becoming more passive; and antidepressant drugs may adversely affect sexual response.

Misunderstanding, ignorance, unsuitable circumstances for having sex, guilt and bad feelings about sex and/or partner can contribute to anxiety and fear of failure, leading to sexual dysfunction.

Inanimate and animate aspects of the environment profoundly affect sexual arousal and response and, of course, determine whether intimate behaviour will take place at all, as well as its efficiency and enjoyability. This includes where and when sex takes place, the ambient temperature, who else is present or nearby, light or darkness, clothing and so forth. Whether particular circumstances are excitatory or inhibitory is largely culturally determined.

> **Biological (both current and developmental), social, cultural, environmental and psychological factors can contribute to sexual dysfunction. All should be considered in each assessment**

Assessing sexual dysfunction

The affected behaviours should be elicited in detail: who is doing what (or wishes to do what), to whom and in what circumstances?

The onset of a problem should be specified. A gradual onset, especially after previously satisfactory sexual activity and with a good concurrent relationship, points to an important physical cause. However, it is often impossible to identify what physical factors are involved. The timing and circumstances of altered sexual interest, and its association with interpersonal conflicts should be noted.

Psychological causes of sexual dysfunctions should be identified positively and not merely by exclusion. Common attributional biases may cloud the issue: women tend to blame themselves for marital difficulties and the sexual complaints of their partners, or to blame their menstrual (or menopausal) status for loss of sexual interest or other difficulties. Both men and women find it easier to blame physical factors (such as medication) for their sexual problems than the much more common conflicts in a relationship or family.

A physical examination is an essential part of the assessment (Box 12.1), but the doctor should be sensitive to its potential emotional impact. It is usually good clinical practice for women patients with sexual complaints to be examined by women.

> ### Box 12.1 **Indications for physical examination**
>
> When physical examination is essential
> - Recent history of ill health, physical or mental
> - Presence of physical symptoms
> - Pain or discomfort during sexual activity
> - Sudden loss of sexual desire without any apparent cause
> - Inability to produce normal erection whilst awake
> - Men over the age of 50
> - Women in perimenopausal groups
> - History of abnormal puberty or endocrine disorder

Investigating sexual dysfunction

Appropriate investigation will depend on the patient's history, and specialist referral may also be considered. If the referrer is almost certain that an important physical factor is relevant referral to a specialist urological, gynaecological or medical clinic may be made. However, when there is any suggestion that psychological factors are involved, then referral to a sexual and relationships clinic, if available, is likely to provide a more comprehensive service.

In cases of erectile failure, intracavernosal injection of papaverine or prostaglandin E1 may be useful initially as an investigation under carefully controlled conditions, and both these drugs can become treatments. Patients with diabetic neuropathy usually respond well to injection, while those with arteriopathic conditions do not.

Treating sexual dysfunction

Treatment involves attention to physical, psychological and social aspects: all should be considered in every case.

An exclusively biological approach without full conversational inquiry is not satisfactory and increases the chance of treatment failure or relapse. Nevertheless, the treatment of impotence has been revolutionised in recent years by the development of improved physical methods, including intracavernosal injections; the use of a vacuum device; various creams and ointments containing nitrite, which may be beneficial when rubbed into the penis; and the operative insertion of semi-rigid rods, which may provide a semi-erection sufficient for coitus.

Newer drugs such as sildenafil, todalafil and vardenafil can be used successfully if the indications are right. These need to be used with caution in patients who have cardiovascular disease. The patient must be advised to take the medication as prescribed and not combine it with complementary or alternative medicine. These drugs are contraindicated in hypotension, recent stroke, unstable angina and myocardial infarction. These are available on NHS prescription under specific conditions.

Psychosocial treatments include general counselling to allow attentive exploration of concerns and specific counselling for the cognitive distortions that may accompany mood problems. Some techniques are derived from the 'Masters and Johnson' approach, which includes non-genital intimacy during an agreed ban on sexual intercourse to alleviate anxiety about performance, and a 'stop-start' approach to improve ejaculatory control. Treatment goals should be agreed that can be approached gradually so as to replace experiences of failure with successes and anxiety with enjoyment. This usually entails practice ('homework') between sessions.

Specific couple therapy may be necessary to treat problems with communication or to enhance a couple's skills in resolving conflict and solving problems. These methods are well suited for use in primary care.

Sexual drive problems

Men and women often have feelings of inferiority about their sexual capacity, but this is not an illness. Loss of (or, less commonly, increase in) sexual drive or interest is common in both men and women. This may manifest in changes in thoughts, fantasies, experienced urges, inclination to initiate sexual activity or specific changes in sexual behaviour. Sometimes in men, the worry about the size of the penis can contribute to performance anxiety as well as lack of desire.

> 'Libido' is a vague term and best avoided. 'Sexual drive' or 'sexual interest' are better terms in clinical practice

Gender problems

Serious problems of gender may accompany endocrinological and developmental disorders that produce ambiguous external genitalia or excessive masculinisation or feminisation.

Transsexualism is a gender identity disorder characterised by a life-long feeling that one's true gender is discordant with one's phenotype. This is associated with an insistent search for gender reassignment procedures, most notably for surgical intervention to make the body more concordant with the experienced self. It affects about one in 700 people and is 10 times more common in men than women. In adults, treatment employs a combination of social, medical and surgical measures to help patients achieve their aims, rather than to try to alter their gender identity. Surgical procedures remain controversial but can produce considerable psychological benefit in selected cases.

Sexual variations and deviations

Paraphilias are problems arising from sexual preferences that are unwelcome to the patients, to others or to society at large. They represent modifications of the capacity for erotic response to another adult and can be understood as a disconnection between sex and affection. Most paraphilias involve behaviours that play a small part in usual adult lovemaking: for example, exposing, sexual looking, dominating, submitting, dressing up and sexual regard for particular objects. In a paraphilia, however, such behaviour becomes the erotic end in itself.

While a range of paraphiliac activities has been described, recurring patterns include sadomasochism (the infliction or experience of pain), transvestism (cross-dressing), fetishism and various illegal activities such as exposing the genitals in public and sexual preference for pre-pubertal children. The assessment and treatment of paraphilias is a specialist matter, especially when the patient presents via the criminal justice system. Psychological treatments are often of considerable value, but the availability of services is very patchy and awareness of local arrangements is essential.

Personal account of mental health problems

Letitcia. *Body worship*. Chipmunkapublishing, Brentwood, Essex, 2006. www.chipmunka.com

Further reading

Semple D, Smyth R, Burns J *et al.* Disorders of behaviour. In: Semple D, Smyth R, Burns J *et al.*, eds *Oxford handbook of psychiatry*. Oxford University Press, Oxford, 2006: 426–37.

CHAPTER 13

Addiction and Dependence: Illicit Drugs

Clare Gerada and Mark Ashworth

OVERVIEW

- Illicit drug misuse is most common in teenage and its prevalence decreases in older people; cannabis is the most abused drug

- Clinical conditions associated with drug misuse are similar for all drugs: acute intoxication, harmful use, dependence, withdrawal and psychosis

- Social and personality factors tend to determine whether someone will misuse drugs; biological effects of the drug, especially euphoria, tend to determine if that person develops dependence

- Medical complications may arise from the biological effects of the drug, its route of administration or the associated lifestyle

- Management of established drug misuse involves general measures to minimise risk of complications, and specific interventions to withdraw the drug or prevent dose escalation

---

Several clinical conditions are recognised as arising from misuse of drugs (Box 13.1). Their clinical features are similar regardless of the drug misused

Why use drugs?

What determines whether drug use becomes continuous and problematic includes:

- Sociocultural factors such as cost, availability and legal status of the drug
- Controls and sanctions on its use
- Age (people in their teens to their 20s are most at risk) and gender (male)
- Peer group of the person taking the drug.

Size of the problem

More than a quarter of the UK population has used an illicit drug in their lifetime, with highest rates found in 16–19-year-olds (46%) and 20–29-year-olds (41%). Use decreases in higher age groups to 12% at 50–59 years. Cannabis is the most commonly used illicit drug and is likely to be taken frequently, with at least 9% of all users reporting daily use. About 100,000 people misuse heroin and an unknown but increasing number use other drugs such as ecstasy and amphetamines. The numbers using crack-cocaine have been increasing since the 1990s and around 2–4% of the population use this drug. Many people stop taking drugs of their own volition and most drug use is largely experimental and transient.

While the number of new drug users continues to rise, the number who inject drugs is falling, possibly as a result of health education about risks of HIV transmission. The highest number of addicts are found in London and the north-west of England, though drug use in rural areas is becoming an increasing problem.

Box 13.1 **Clinical conditions associated with drug misuse**

Acute intoxication: may be uncomplicated or associated with bodily injury, delirium, convulsions or coma. Includes 'bad trips' due to hallucinogenic drugs

Harmful use: a pattern of drug misuse resulting in physical harm (such as hepatitis) or mental harm (such as depression) to the user. These consequences often elicit negative reactions from other people and result in social disruption for the user

Dependence syndrome: obtaining and using the drug assume the highest priorities in the user's life. A person may be dependent on a single substance (such as diazepam), a group of related drugs (such as the opioids) or a wide range of different drugs. This is the state known colloquially as drug addiction

Withdrawal: usually occurs when a patient is abstinent after a prolonged period of drug use, especially if large doses were used. Withdrawal is time-limited, but withdrawal may cause convulsions and require medical treatment

Psychotic disorder: many drugs can produce the hallucinations, delusions and behavioural disturbances characteristic of psychosis. Patterns of symptoms may be extremely variable, even during a single episode. Early onset syndromes (within 48 hours) may mimic schizophrenia or psychotic depression; late-onset syndromes (after two weeks or more) include flashbacks, personality changes and cognitive deterioration

ABC of Mental Health, 2nd edition. Edited by T. Davies and T. Craig. © 2009 Blackwell Publishing, ISBN: 978-0-7279-1639-6.

Personality factors determine how a person copes once addicted and the mechanisms he or she may use to seek help. A number of protective factors are recognised:

- Consistent parenting
- Scholastic achievement
- Involvement in sporting or other hobbies
- Responsibilities such as managing a home.

Commonly misused drugs

> Common drugs of misuse tend to cause euphoria and dependence

Benzodiazepines

Though not strictly speaking illicit (illegal) benzodiazepines are subject to abuse. Benzodiazepines are almost invariably misused alongside heroin and cocaine, often in very large doses (for example, several 100 mg diazepam-equivalents per day). Reasons for use are multifold and sometimes contradictory. They include to 'get high', to offset the stimulant effects of cocaine or to prolong the hedonistic effects of heroin. This group of users should be differentiated from those with long-term iatrogenic dependence. This latter group tend to be elderly and use much lower doses initially prescribed as an anxiolytic or hypnotic.

A withdrawal syndrome can occur after only three weeks of continuous use, and it affects a third of long-term users. The syndrome usually consists of increased anxiety and perceptual disturbances, especially heightened sensitivity to light and sound; occasionally there are fits, hallucinations and confusion. Depending on the drug's half-life, symptoms start one to five days after the last dose, peak within 10 days, and subside after one to six weeks.

Opioids

Opioids (the term includes naturally occurring opiates such as heroin and opium and synthetic opiates such as pethidine and methadone) produce an intense but transient feeling of pleasure. Withdrawal symptoms begin a few hours from the last dose, peak after two to three days and subside after a week (Box 13.2). Heroin is available in a powdered form, commonly mixed ('cut') with other substances such as chalk or lactose powder. It can be sniffed ('snorting'), eaten, smoked ('chasing the dragon'), injected subcutaneously ('skin popping') or injected intravenously ('mainlining'). Tablets can be crushed and then injected.

> Box 13.2 **Heroin withdrawal syndrome**
>
> - Insomnia
> - Muscle pains and cramps
> - Increased salivary, nasal and lachrymal secretions
> - Anorexia, nausea, vomiting and diarrhoea
> - Dilated pupils
> - Yawning

Amphetamines

These cause generalised over-arousal with hyperactivity, tachycardia, dilated pupils and fine tremor. Effects last about three to four hours, after which the user becomes tired, anxious, irritable and restless. High doses and chronic use can produce psychosis with paranoid delusions, hallucinations and over-activity. Physical dependence can occur, and termination of prolonged use may cause profound depression and lassitude. Amphetamines were widely prescribed in the 1960s: the most common current source is illegally produced amphetamine sulphate powder, which can be taken by mouth, by sniffing or by intravenous injection. Metamphetamine ('ice', 'crystal', 'glass') is chemically related to amphetamine but has more potent effects. It is associated with severe mental health problems.

Cocaine

Cocaine preparations can be eaten (coca leaves or paste), injected alone or with heroin ('speedballing'), sniffed ('snow') or smoked (as 'crack'). Crack is cocaine in its base form and is smoked because of the speed and intensity of its psychoactive effects. The stimulant effect ('rush') is felt within seconds of smoking crack, peaks in one to five minutes and wears off after about 15 minutes.

Smokable cocaine produces physical dependence with craving: the withdrawal state is characterised by depression and lethargy followed by increased craving, which can last up to three months. Use by any route can result in death from myocardial infarction, hyperthermia or ventricular arrhythmias. Around one-quarter of myocardial infarcts in young adults (those under 45 years) are caused by cocaine use.

Ecstasy (3,4-methylenedioxymethamphetamine, MDMA)

An increasingly popular drug, especially at 'rave' parties, ecstasy (known as 'E') has hallucinogenic properties and produces euphoria and increased energy. Continuous or excessive use with raised physical activity can lead to hyperthermia and dehydration with the risk of sudden death (although attempts at preventing dehydration by encouraging consumption of large quantities of water risks producing hyponatraemic seizures).

Cannabis

There are over 1000 different forms of cannabis ranging from herbal varieties (marijuana, 'bush', 'grass', 'weed', 'draw'), home-grown varieties ('skunk', 'northern lights') and resins ('soap bar', accounting for roughly two-thirds of UK consumption and typically combined with plastic, diesel to aid combustion and henna for colour). Cannabis is most commonly smoked and it is in this form that it causes most harm to the lungs (lung cancer, bronchitis, asthma) and mental health problems (anxiety, paranoia, psychosis). Tar from cannabis contains up to 50% higher concentrations of carcinogens than tobacco smoke. There is some evidence that the potency of certain types of cannabis has increased in recent years. The effects of cannabis are dose-related, and, hence, any change in strength is important. Around 5–10% of regular users develop dependence characterised by craving and withdrawal symptoms.

Misused volatile substances

Such substances include glues (the most common), gas fuels, cleaning agents, correcting fluid thinners and aerosols. Their main misuse is among young boys as part of a group activity; those who misuse alone tend to be more disturbed and in need of psychiatric help. Their effects are similar to alcohol: intoxication with initial euphoria followed by disorientation, blurred vision, dizziness, slurred speech, ataxia and drowsiness. About 100 people die each year from misusing volatile substances, mainly from direct toxic effects.

Dependence syndrome

The dependence syndrome is a cluster of symptoms, not all of which need be present for a diagnosis of dependence to be made. The key feature is a compulsion to use drugs, which results in overwhelming priority being given to drug-seeking behaviour. Other features are tolerance (need to increase drug dose to achieve desired effect), withdrawal (both physical and psychological symptoms on stopping use) and use of drug to relieve or avoid withdrawal symptoms. An addict's increasing focus on drug-seeking behaviour leads to progressive loss of other interests, neglect of self-care and social relationships, and disregard for harmful consequences. The term 'addiction' implies that the drug has a strong propensity to produce dependence. Highly addictive drugs tend to have the ability to produce intensely pleasurable effects.

Medical complications of drug misuse

Complications can arise secondary to the drug used (such as constipation), route of drug use (such as deep vein thrombosis) and the lifestyle associated with a drug habit (such as self-neglect, crime). Complications commonly arise from injecting drugs (Box 13.3): using dirty and non-sterile needles risks cellulitis, endocarditis and septicaemia; sharing injecting equipment ('works') can transmit HIV, hepatitis B and hepatitis C; and incorrect technique and injecting impurities can result in venous thrombosis or accidental arterial puncture.

Box 13.3 **Complications of injecting drug use**

Poor injecting technique
- Abscess
- Cellulitis
- Thrombophlebitis
- Arterial puncture
- Deep vein thrombosis

Needle sharing
- Hepatitis B and C
- HIV or AIDS

Drug content or contaminants
- Abscess
- Overdose
- Gangrene
- Thrombosis

Box 13.4 **Important interactions between illicit and prescribed drugs**

Amphetamines
- Antipsychotics: antipsychotic effects opposed. Euphoric effects of amphetamines reduced, so misuse increased to compensate
- Mood stabilisers: carbamazepine may result in hepatotoxic metabolites
- Monoamine oxidase inhibitors: potentially fatal hypertensive crisis
- Tricyclic antidepressants: arrhythmias

Cannabis
- Antipsychotics: antipsychotic effects opposed. Euphoric effects reduced, so misuse increased to compensate
- Fluoxetine: increased energy, hypersexuality, pressured speech
- Tricyclic antidepressants: marked tachycardia

Cocaine
- Monoamine oxidase inhibitors: possibility of hypertension

Ecstasy
- Antipsychotics: more prone to extrapyramidal side effects
- Monoamine oxidase inhibitors: hypertension

Opioids
- Antipsychotics: euphoric effects reduced, so misuse increased to compensate
- Desipramine: methadone doubles serum levels of desipramine
- Diazepam: increased central nervous system depression
- Mood stabilisers: carbamazepine reduces methadone levels
- Monoamine oxidase inhibitors: potentially fatal interaction with pethidine

---

A major hazard of intravenous misuse is overdose, which may be accidental or deliberate (Box 13.4). Death from intravenous opioid overdose can be rapid. Opioid overdose should be suspected in any unconscious patient, especially in combination with pinpoint pupils and respiratory depression. Immediate injection of the opioid antagonist naloxone can be lifesaving. Cannabis can increase the risk of developing lung cancer and other respiratory problems, such as asthma.

Practical management

General principles
Management ranges from steps to prevent drug misuse in individuals and groups, through risk minimisation, to specific interventions focused on the individual patient and the drug being misused.
- Prevent misuse by careful prescribing of potential drugs of misuse such as analgesics, hypnotics and tranquillisers
- Encourage patients into treatment and help them to remain in contact with services
- Reduce harm associated with drug use
- Treat physical complications of drug use and interactions with prescribed drugs
- Offer general medical care (such as hepatitis immunisation and cervical screening)
- Offer effective evidence-based psychological and pharmacological interventions.

> **Box 13.5 Factors to be recorded in a drug assessment**
>
> **Drug taken**
> - Opioids: heroin, methadone, buprenorphine, dihydrocodeine (DF118), others
> - Benzodiazepines
> - Stimulants: cocaine, amphetamines, ecstasy, others
> - Alcohol
> - Cannabis
>
> **For each drug**
> - Amount taken: in weight (g), cost (£), volume (mL), number of tablets, units of alcohol
> - How often: daily, intermittently, clubbing, raves
> - Route of administration: intravenous, intramuscular, subcutaneous, oral, inhaled

Specific measures

The full drug history must include all substances taken, duration and frequency of use, amount of drug used (recorded verbatim, including amount spent daily on drugs) and route of drug use (Box 13.5). Do not forget to ask about alcohol consumption as many drug users are also heavy consumers of alcohol.

Injecting users will have needle track marks, usually in the antecubital fossae, although any venous site can be used. Further investigation should include a (fresh) urine drug screen and contacting previous prescribing doctors or dispensing pharmacists to confirm history.

Withdrawal from non-opioid drugs

To withdraw a patient from any benzodiazepine, first convert the misused drug into an equivalent dose of diazepam, chosen because of its long half-life. Reduce the diazepam dose by 2 mg a fortnight over a period of two to six months. Even those individuals on large amounts of benzodiazepines can be reduced fairly rapidly. For a small minority of patients, a maintenance prescription of benzodiazepines may be more beneficial than insisting on abstinence. This is best undertaken in collaboration with a specialist service.

At present there is no recommended substitution treatment for cocaine or amphetamines, although many different pharmacological treatments have been tried. Antidepressants in therapeutic doses may help specific symptoms. Cannabis, ecstasy and volatile (solvent) substances may all be withdrawn abruptly, but abstinence is more likely to be maintained if attention is paid to any psychological symptoms that emerge. Nicotine cessation products may be a helpful adjunct in cannabis withdrawal to offset any nicotine withdrawal effects.

Treating opioid dependence

Maintenance, either with methadone mixture (1 mg/mL) or buprenorphine should be the mainstay of management for opioid dependence, certainly until the patient is able and willing to withdraw ('detoxify') and achieve abstinence. Methadone maintenance treatment has been shown to be effective in reducing health, criminal and social harms in trials, including many randomised, double-blind studies.

> **Any doctor in the UK can prescribe methadone or buprenorphine**

Methadone

Before prescribing, it is important first to establish the diagnosis of dependence (as above), and second to understand the risks inherent in inducing patients on to methadone. Methadone, in doses as low as 30–40 mg, can be fatal in naïve users. General advice when starting someone on methadone is to start low (10–20 mg) per day and increase the dose gradually (5–10 mg/day) over the following 7–14 days until the patient is comfortable, in that they are neither intoxicated nor suffering from withdrawal. Research now suggests that there should be no ceiling dose of methadone, and that higher doses (60–120 mg/day) are associated with better outcome than lower ones. Any clinician who is not familiar with methadone treatment should ensure that they are supported by shared care (community nurse, general practitioner with special interest or addiction specialist). In summary:

- Be safe
- Establish the diagnosis of opiate dependence (history, examination, urine test)
- Confirm dependence (daily or frequent use, craving and withdrawal on cessation)
- Start low – go slow.

Buprenorphine

This partial agonist/antagonist is a useful new addition to the treatment armoury of opioid dependence. As with methadone, a careful assessment and diagnosis of dependence should be the first step before prescribing. Buprenorphine can be used for detoxification or maintenance as with methadone, research suggests that higher (12–14 mg/day) rather than lower maintenance doses are associated with better outcome. Induction onto buprenorphine can be achieved over a number of days; starting at a dose between 2 and 4 mg, increasing by 2–4 mg/day until stable. The clinician should specifically request a buprenorphine assay when monitoring compliance with urine tests.

How to prescribe opioids

General practitioners may use blue FP10 (MDA) prescriptions, which allow daily instalments on a single prescription, thus reducing the risk of overdose or diversion into the black market. Prescriptions for controlled drugs must:

- Be written in indelible ink
- Be signed and dated by the doctor
- State the form and strength of the preparation
- State doses in words and figures
- State the total dose
- Specify the amount in each instalment and the intervals between instalments.

Doctors granted Home Office Handwriting Dispensation can issue computer-generated prescriptions, but still need to sign and date the prescription in their own hand.

Further information

British Doctors' and Dentists' Group (Independent self help organisation for alcohol and drug dependent doctors and dentists). Contacted via Medical Council on Alcohol, tel. 020 7487 4445. http://www.medicouncilalcol.demon.co.uk/

Narcotics Anonymous, tel. 020 7730 0009, http://www.ukna.org/

Further reading

Department of Health, The Scottish Office Department of Health, Welsh Office, Department of Health and Social Security in Northern Ireland. *Drug misuse and dependence – Guidelines on clinical management*. The Stationery Office, London, 1999. www.dh.gov.uk/en/Policyandguidance/Healthandsocialcaretopics/Substancemisuse/AtoZofSubstanceMisuseGuidancePublications/index.htm?indexChar=D

Gerada C, Joyhns K, Baker A, Castle D. Substance use and abuse in women. In: Castle D, Kulkarni J, Abel KM eds. *Mood and anxiety disorders in women*. Cambridge University Press, Cambridge, 2006.

Haslam D, Beaumont B. *Care of drug users in general practice. A harm reduction approach*, 2nd edn. Radcliffe Publishing, Oxford, 2004.

Keen J. Methadone maintenance prescribing, how to get the best results. http://www.smmgp.org.uk

National Institute for Health and Clinical Excellence. *Drug misuse: Psychosocial interventions*. NICE guideline CG51. NICE, London, 2007. http://guidance.nice.org.uk/CG51/

National Institute for Health and Clinical Excellence. *Drug misuse: Opioid detoxification*. NICE guideline CG52. NICE, London, 2007. http://guidance.nice.org.uk/CG52/

Royal College of General Practitioners. *Guidance for the use of buprenorphine for the treatment of opioid dependence in primary care*. RCGP, London, 2004. Obtainable from RCGP Substance Misuse Unit, 314 Frazer House, 32–38 Leman Street, London, E1 8EW. http://www.smmgp.org.uk/html/guidance.php

Seivewright N. *Community treatment of drug misuse: More than methadone*. Cambridge University Press, Cambridge, 2000.

CHAPTER 14

Addiction and Dependence: Alcohol

Mark Ashworth, Clare Gerada and Yvonne Doyle

OVERVIEW

- Recommended upper limits of alcohol consumption (21 units a week for men and 14 units for women) are exceeded by about 29% of men and 17% of women in the UK

- Problem drinking may be detected in about 75% of cases by the Alcohol Use Disorders Identification Test (AUDIT) supplemented by blood tests for mean corpuscular volume (MCV) and gamma-glutamyl transferase (GGT)

- Controlled withdrawal of alcohol may take place in the community with benzodiazepine attenuation therapy; but inpatient withdrawal is recommended for those at risk of suicide or severe withdrawal reactions

- Delirium tremens occurs in about 5% of those withdrawing from alcohol about 48–72 hours or more after the last drink; this is a medical emergency with over 10% mortality

- Relapse rate among dependent drinkers is high but can be reduced by a programme of rehabilitation

---

Prevalence of alcohol-related problems

As with any drug of addiction, there are four levels of alcohol use.

1 Social drinking: only about 10% of the population are teetotal.
2 At risk consumption: this is the level of alcohol intake that, if maintained, poses a risk to health (Box 14.1). *The Health of the Nation* gives 'safe' levels of consumption as 21 units a week for men and 14 units a week for women. According to the UK General Household Survey, these levels are exceeded by a sizeable minority of the population – 29% of men and 17% of women; almost 4% of the population regularly drink in excess of double these limits. More recently, the emphasis on limits for weekly consumption has changed because of increased awareness of the dangers of binge drinking. Instead, safe limits are now expressed as daily maximums: three to four units for men and two to three units for women. Even these limits come with the caveat that continued consumption at the upper level is not advised. Increased awareness of the dangers of foetal damage attributable to maternal alcohol consumption (foetal alcohol syndrome

---

Box 14.1 **Alcohol-related problems**

- 18,500 deaths a year in England and Wales are related to alcohol consumption
- 300 of these deaths are the direct result of alcoholic liver damage (the true figure is probably many times higher but is hidden by under-reporting on death certificates)
- Just over 1 in 1000 people die per year of an alcohol-related problem

Alcohol consumption is associated with:
- 80% of suicides
- 50% of murders
- 50% of violent crimes
- 80% of deaths from fire
- 40% of road traffic accidents
- 30% of fatal road traffic accidents
- 15% of drownings

Alcohol consumption contributes to:
- One in three divorces
- One in three cases of child abuse
- 20–30% of all hospital admissions

Data from *Alcohol related death rates in England and Wales, 2001–2003*. Office of National Statistics, London, 2005.

---

and neurocognitive defects such as hyperactivity and impulsive behaviour) has resulted in recommendations that pregnant women should drink little or nothing at all.

> **Alcohol exacts a huge toll on the nation's physical, social and psychological health. Consumption doubled between 1950 and 1980, during which time the relative price of alcohol halved. Since then consumption has flattened off**

3 Problem drinking: at this level, consumption causes serious problems to drinkers, their family and social network, or to society. About 1–2% of the population have alcohol problems.
4 Dependence and addiction: the characteristics of dependence apply to alcohol as to other drugs – periodic or chronic intoxication, uncontrollable craving, tolerance resulting in dose increase, dependence (either psychological or physical), and a detrimental result to the person or society. There are about 200,000 dependent drinkers in the United Kingdom.

ABC of Mental Health, 2nd edition. Edited by T. Davies and T. Craig.
© 2009 Blackwell Publishing, ISBN: 978-0-7279-1639-6.

Binge drinking is an increasing phenomenon, predominantly occurring in the under 25s. It is defined as drinking eight or more units for males and six or more units for females on a single occasion. Rates for young women are rising rapidly. Currently, about 4 million men and 1.9 million women report binge drinking in the past week.

Factors affecting consumption

Consumption of alcohol depends on several variables.

- Sex: although men are twice as likely to have alcohol-related problems, the gap between the sexes is narrowing
- Occupation: alcohol misuse is more common in jobs related to catering, brewing and distilling. In others, such as doctors, sailors and demolition workers, high consumption may be perceived as the social norm
- Homelessness: about a third of homeless people have alcohol problems
- Race: about a fifth of Chinese and Japanese people cannot drink alcohol because of an inherited lack of the liver enzyme acetaldehyde dehydrogenase

---

People lacking the liver enzyme acetaldehyde dehydrogenase experience extremely unpleasant reactions on exposure to alcohol because of accumulation of acetaldehyde. Reactions include nausea, flushing, headache, palpitations and collapse. Alcohol evokes a similar response in patients who are given disulfiram

---

Recognising problem drinking

Recognising people with alcohol-related problems is difficult – probably less than 20% are known to their general practitioner (although problem drinkers consult their GP twice as frequently as those whose alcohol consumption is within the safe limits), and a large proportion are missed in accident and emergency departments. Recognition is particularly difficult among teenagers, elderly people and doctors. About half of the doctors reported to the General Medical Council for health difficulties liable to affect professional competence have an alcohol problem.

Doctors may be alerted to an alcohol problem by the presenting complaint. The essential first stage in improving recognition is taking a drinking history, and this should be combined with selected investigations.

- Amount of alcohol consumed in units. Always enquire about quantity and type of drink. Many doctors are unaware of the unit values for common descriptions of daily intake (Box 14.2)
- Time of first alcoholic drink of the day
- Pattern of drinking: problem drinking is characterised by the establishment of an unvarying pattern of daily drinking
- Presence of withdrawal symptoms such as early morning shakes or nausea.

Specific questioning should follow the World Health Organization's Alcohol Use Disorders Identification Test (AUDIT), which includes questions from the well-known CAGE questionnaire (Box 14.3).

Box 14.2 **Estimating alcohol consumption as units**

One unit is equivalent to 10 mL alcohol. To calculate the number of units in any alcoholic drink, multiply the volume in mL by the strength (% alcohol by volume, ABV) and divide the total by 1000.

Alcohol consumption may be underestimated if calculated using traditional measures and strengths. So, for example, one unit of alcohol is contained in 1/2 pint (284 mL) of 3.5% strength beer, one small glass (125 mL) of 9% strength wine, or one measure (25 mL) of 40% spirits.

Whilst the definition of a unit has not changed, both the strength and size of commonly sold alcoholic drinks has increased.

- Beer is usually stronger than 3.5% ABV. A 330 mL bottle of 4% beer contains one and a half units. A large can of strong lager (500 mL at 8% ABV) contains four units
- Wine is usually stronger than 9% and often served in larger glasses. More typically, a 12% strength wine in a 175 mL glass contains 2.1 units
- Spirits: pub measures are more usually 35 mL resulting in a measure of spirits containing 1.4 units

---

Box 14.3 **CAGE questionnaire**

Alcohol dependence is likely if the patient gives two or more positive answers to the following questions:

- Have you ever felt you should **C**ut down on your drinking?
- Have people **A**nnoyed you by criticising your drinking?
- Have you ever felt bad or **G**uilty about your drinking?
- Have you ever had a drink first thing in the morning to steady your nerves or get rid of hangover (**E**ye-opener)?

Ewing JA. Detecting alcoholism – the CAGE questionnaire. *JAMA* 1984; **252**: 1905–7.

Investigation should include measuring the mean corpuscular volume (MCV) and gamma-glutamyl transferase (GGT) activity. This combination of tests will detect about 75% of people with an alcohol problem, while measuring GGT alone detects only a third of cases (Box 14.4).

Managing alcohol dependence

Detoxification

Alcohol dependence usually requires controlled withdrawal (detoxification) with an attenuation therapy (such as a benzodiazepine), as abrupt cessation of alcohol can induce one of the withdrawal states (Box 14.5). Detoxification is increasingly taking place in the community, but inpatient detoxification is recommended for those at risk of suicide, lacking social support or giving a history of severe withdrawal reactions including fits and delirium tremens.

About a third of people who seriously misuse alcohol recover without any professional intervention

The important principles of community detoxification are:
- Daily supervision in order to allow early detection of complications such as delirium tremens, continuous vomiting or deterioration in mental state (confusion or drowsiness)
- The vitamin B preparation, thiamine 50 mg twice daily for three weeks, is needed to prevent Wernicke's encephalopathy. This should be given to all patients undergoing withdrawal. Severely alcohol-dependent patients will need initial treatment with parenteral vitamins (such as Pabrinex™), which, because of the risk of anaphylaxis, makes this category of patients unsuitable for a community detoxification
- Benzodiazepines to prevent a withdrawal syndrome. Because of the potential for dependence, benzodiazepines should be prescribed for a limited period only. The most commonly used benzodiazepine is chlordiazepoxide at a starting dose of 10 mg four times daily and reducing over seven days. Larger doses are used in severe withdrawal – for example, 40 mg four times daily reducing over 14 days. On the other hand, large doses may accumulate to dangerous levels if there is significant liver disease, and, in these circumstances, oxazepam is preferred.

Support after withdrawal

The relapse rate among alcoholics is high, but can be reduced by a programme of rehabilitation. Various options are available to assist in maintaining recovery:
- Primary healthcare team
- Community alcohol team
- Residential rehabilitation programmes
- Voluntary organisations providing support and counselling, either individually or in groups (Box 14.6)
- Supervised medication regimens (see below)
- Referral to specialist mental health services for patients who show substantial psychiatric comorbidity. An important subgroup of alcoholics will require treatment for phobic anxiety or recurrent depression.

Medication

Disulfiram has a small but useful role to play in maintaining abstinence. Patients who take disulfiram (which inhibits acetaldehyde dehydrogenase) experience the extremely unpleasant symptoms of acetaldehyde accumulation if they drink any alcohol; although usually this takes the form of vomiting, the reaction can be unpredictable and severe reactions can occur, causing collapse and requiring oxygen treatment. Controlled studies show that supervised administration (by relatives, doctors or primary care staff), either alone or as an adjunct to psychosocial methods, is one of the few effective interventions in alcohol dependence. Abstinence rates approaching 60% at one year have been reported.

Disulfiram treatment should not be started unless the patient has been alcohol-free for 24 hours. Caution is also required about unwitting alcohol consumption during treatment – for example, alcohol contained in cough medicines, tonics and foods. Even after stopping disulfiram, the patient should avoid alcohol for at least one week. Disulfiram should not be given to patients with active liver disease, cardiovascular disorders, suicidal risk or cognitive impairment. There is no limit on the duration of disulfiram treatment, but liver function tests should be checked at six months as the drug itself may cause liver damage. It is contraindicated if liver disease is severe (liver enzymes over ten times normal limits).

Acamprosate is licensed for use in alcohol dependence. It acts to reduce craving for alcohol probably through a direct effect on GABA receptors in the brain; unlike disulfiram it produces no adverse interaction with alcohol and so has no deterrent effect. It is a useful alternative in maintaining abstinence. It is recommended that treatment is started as soon as possible after detoxification and should be maintained even in the event of a relapse. The recommended duration of treatment is one year. Continued alcohol abuse cancels out any therapeutic benefit and treatment should then be stopped. Like disulfiram, it is contraindicated in severe liver disease.

Personal account of mental health problems

Spiegler E. *Missing mummy. Living in the shadow of an alcoholic parent.* Chipmunkapublishing, Brentwood, Essex, 2006. www.chipmunka.com

Further reading

Babor TF, Higgins-Biddle JC, Saunders JB, Monteiro MG. *The alcohol use disorders identification test. Guidelines for use in primary care*, 2nd edn. World Health Organization, Geneva, 2001.

Cabinet Office, Prime Minister's Strategy Unit. *Alcohol harm reduction strategy for England*. Cabinet Office, London, 2004. http://www.strategy.gov.uk/su/alcohol/pdf/CabOffce%20AlcoholHar.pdf

Edwards G, Marshall EJ, Cook CCH. *The treatment of drinking problems.* Cambridge University Press, Cambridge, 2003.

Miller WR, Rollnick S. *Motivational interviewing: Preparing people for change*, 2nd edn. Guilford Publications, New York, 2002.

UK Alcohol Forum. *Guidelines for the management of alcohol problems in primary care and general psychiatry*, 1997. www.ukalcoholforum.org/

Williams H, Ghodse H. The prevention of alcohol and drug misuse. In: Kendrick T, Tylee A, Freeling P, eds. *The prevention of mental illness in primary care.* Cambridge University Press, Cambridge, 1996: 223–45.

Mental Health Problems in Old Age

Chris Ball

The health service has changed apace since the first edition of this *ABC*. Top-down management of services has made sweeping changes in the mental health services for adult's of working age, achieved with (from an older adult's perspective) massive financial investment. Older adults mental health services have also had to change, responding to 'high level drivers', developments in treatment options and increasingly close work with other agencies both statutory and non-statutory. For the most part these have been changes for the better, but the failure to fund the National Service Framework (NSF) for Older People, and the pressure on NHS trusts to meet the milestones of the NSF for adults of working age, have often left older adults' services at a disadvantage. However, older adults' services seem to be increasingly important on the political agenda, and there are hopes that these important services can be put on a sound footing, to help address the very extensive suffering that mental health problems bring to the elderly population.

Depression

Depression is common but not inevitable with ageing (Box 15.1). The assumption that being old must be a miserable experience colours the judgement of many healthcare professionals and older

ABC of Mental Health, 2nd edition. Edited by T. Davies and T. Craig.
© 2009 Blackwell Publishing, ISBN: 978-0-7279-1639-6.

Box 15.1 **Prevalence of depression among people over 65**

General community	15%
General practice attendees	25%
Residential and nursing homes	45%

adults themselves. What can be expected when you develop physical problems, your friends and family are dying, and you can no longer do all the things you used to do?

The problem with this attitude is that depression is regarded as the normal response to such circumstances. Whilst you might be sympathetic there is no other intervention for a normal response. This leads to under-recognition and under-treatment of the disorder.

Recognition

Depression may present in the classic ways with lower mood and lack of interest and energy, but can also present in a number of unusual ways in older adults that cause diagnostic problems. When encountering these presentations, depression should be considered (Box 15.2).

One of the most common associations with depression is the presence of physical illness (Box 15.3). On medical wards, the prevalence is between 11% and 59% depending upon the screening instrument, type of ward surveyed and the sex and age of subjects.

Recognition in these circumstances can be difficult, but to be physically unwell and depressed increases length of stay, delays recovery and impacts upon mortality, particularly in cardio-vascular disorders. Healthcare workers should not be afraid to ask

Box 15.2 **Problems diagnosing depression in older adults**

- Overlap of physical and somatic psychiatric symptoms
- Minimal expression of sadness
- Somatisation
- Deliberate self-harm (infrequent)
- Pseudodementia (memory problems)
- Late-onset alcohol abuse
- Behavioural change

about suicidal ideas. Enquiry is not likely to induce suicide and it is usually a relief for the person to be able to talk about these frightening thoughts.

Management
Psychological

NICE guidelines recommend a 'stepped care' approach to the management of depression that is applicable across the entire adult age range. Highlighting the role of talking therapies is to be welcomed and there is good evidence (particularly for cognitive behavioural therapy, CBT) that age is no barrier to their effectiveness. These therapies are often not considered for elderly people, perhaps because the availability of therapists to undertake this work across the age range is limited.

Social

Small interventions to re-engage people with their community, e.g. provision of transport to their clubs or meetings, can be vitally important for many people.

Medical

Doctors should consider physical illnesses or their treatments that might mimic or induce depression and seek to treat these or modify existing treatment regimens. Treatment with antidepressants has become more straightforward over recent years (Box 15.4), with the improving side effect profile of antidepressant drugs.

Selective serotonin reuptake inhibitors (SSRIs) are first choice treatments (e.g. citalopram, fluoxetine). Once-a-day dosage, relatively cardiac-friendly side effect profile, and low levels of drug interactions make them easy to use. Recent concerns over cardiac toxicity with venlafaxine have tended to limit its use to secondary

care, with a careful evaluation of the risk/benefit profile and ECG monitoring.

A number of other once-a-day medications with acceptable side effect profiles (e.g. mirtazapine or duloxetine) could also be considered. Once the person has recovered from their illness, medication should be continued for at least two years as the time course to full remission can be more prolonged than in younger adults.

Referral

The NSF for Older People identified a number of indications for referral of older adults with depression to secondary services:
- Failure of first-line management
- Doubt about the diagnosis
- Presence of psychosis
- Suicide risk.

Referral should be considered if the patient is not eating and drinking even if the above indications are not met.

Anxiety disorders

Anxiety disorders are as common in older adults as they are in younger populations (10–15%) with substantial numbers presenting to primary care (10–18%).

There is evidence that anxiety disorders are recognised and treated even less often than depression, with the physiological symptoms (Box 15.5) being frequently over-investigated.

Generalised anxiety disorder and specific phobias are the commonest anxiety disorders beginning over the age of 65 (Figure 15.1), and are associated with significantly impaired quality of life. Panic disorder usually runs a chronic course with an early onset. New cases are unusual in late life. Post-traumatic stress disorder (PTSD) is increasingly recognised, with some evidence that symptoms may worsen later in life. Rates of PTSD for young and old following natural disasters are probably the same.

As with depression, there is an association with physical illnesses that may mimic the illness (e.g. hyperthyroidism, alcohol abuse), or be the result of the insecurities engendered by the illness (e.g. falls, chronic obstructive pulmonary disease), or reflect the perceptions of society. Comorbidity with depression is as common as in younger adults, but the impact is greater on quality of life.

Management

NICE guidelines for the management of anxiety have similar steps to those for depression. There is good evidence for the effectiveness

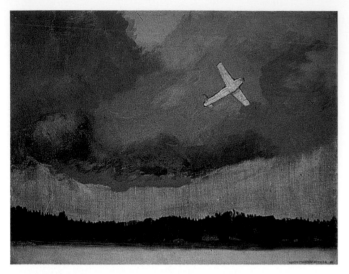

Figure 15.1 Older people have a greater fear of flying than younger people.

of psychological therapies for anxiety in older adults (e.g. CBT), but it is questionable if the resources are available to deliver the care required.

Medical management

Many different compounds have been used for anxiety over the years. The best evidence for effectiveness lies with the SSRIs (e.g. citalopram, fluoxetine) and SNRIs (e.g. venlafaxine). The slow onset of action of these drugs has been a cause for non-concordance, particularly as an initial worsening in symptoms is seen. Education and support through this time is important but some need additional medication to tide them over this brief period.

Benzodiazepines have been used for many years but are recommended for short-term use only. They are particularly problematic with the elderly (Box 15.6), but for the occasional person the only way to have a reasonable quality of life is long-term use. The risks and benefits must always be discussed carefully and recorded in such a case.

Paranoid disorders in the elderly

Late-onset paranoid disorders are relatively rare in older adults (point prevalence 0.1–1.5%), but they consume a great deal of the time and resources of mental health services for older people.

Box 15.6 Problems with benzodiazepine use in older adults

- Drowsiness
- Cognitive impairment
- Psychomotor impairment
- Falls
- Depression
- Amnesic syndromes
- Respiratory depression

Box 15.7 Symptoms in very late-onset schizophrenia

Hallucinations

Auditory	70% non-verbal
	50% third-person voices
	50% second-person voices
Visual	40%
Olfactory	30%

Delusions

Persecution	85%
Reference	75%
Misinterpretation or misidentification	60%
Body/mind control	30%

Rarely presenting in their own right, they are seen by housing officers, by the police and by social workers, and it is rarely recognised that the person might have a mental health problem. When elderly people present with psychotic symptoms, a paranoid disorder is not top of the diagnostic list: the most likely diagnosis is a dementing illness with or without a delirium. A careful history of the psychotic symptoms (acute versus chronic), changes in physical function and cognitive function, should clarify the issue.

Classification of these illnesses has been difficult as often they do not meet the ICD-10 criteria for schizophrenia, nor do they sit comfortably as persistent delusional disorders as hallucinations can be florid. Those with late-onset psychotic disorders are unlikely to experience formal thought disorder or have the negative symptoms seen in early onset cases.

The International Late Onset Schizophrenia Group has proposed the following classification for these schizophrenia-like illnesses: under 40 years of age – schizophrenia; 40–60 years of age – late-onset schizophrenia; and 60+ years of age – very late-onset schizophrenia (Box 15.7).

Management

Engagement with this group can be particularly difficult. Although they see no need for involvement of mental health services – demanding that the police, housing or toxicology services deal with their problems – a sympathetic listener is often welcomed. Common ground should be sought upon which trust can be developed (sorting out financial difficulties, helping with social care, helping to explore some other interest with community groups, dealing with loss). This helps to develop the relationship so that treatment can be initiated. Assessing risk can be difficult as such people can be a nuisance but not dangerous. Where the risks are not sustainable, detention and treatment under the Mental Health Act must be used.

Often there are clear benefits from treatment, with between a third and a half of sufferers responding well to medication (i.e. free of delusions and hallucinations). This seems to be the case with both typical and atypical antipsychotics. Depot medication needs to be considered for those who are unwilling or unable to accept oral medication.

Further reading

Appleby L, Philp I. *Securing better mental health services for older people*. Department of Health, London, 2005. www.dh.gov.uk/PolicyAndGuidance/HealthAndSocialCareTopics/OlderPeoplesServices/fs/en

Department of Health. *National Service Framework for Older People*. DH, London, 2001. http://www.dh.gov.uk/en/Publicationsandstatistics/Publications/PublicationsPolicyAndGuidance/DH_4003066

Garner J, Sibisi C. An open letter from the Faculty of Old Age Psychiatry to Professor Louis Appleby and Professor Ian Philp. *Old Age Psychiatrist* 2005; **39:** 2–3.

Howard R, Rabins PV, Castle DJ, eds. *Late onset schizophrenia*. Wrightson Biomedical Publishing, Petersfield, 1999.

Marriott H. *The selfish pig's guide to caring*. Time Warner, London, 2006.

Mozley CG, Challis D, Sutcliffe C, *et al*. Psychiatric symptomatology in elderly people admitted to nursing and residential homes. *Aging Mental Health* **4:** 136–41.

National Institute for Health and Clinical Excellence. *Schizophrenia: Core interventions in the treatment and management of schizophrenia in primary and secondary care*. NICE guideline CG1. NICE, London, 2002. http://guidance.nice.org.uk/CG1/

National Institute for Health and Clinical Excellence. *Anxiety (amended): Management of anxiety (panic disorder, with or without agoraphobia, and generalised anxiety disorder) in adults in primary, secondary and community care*. NICE guideline CG22, NICE, London, 2007. http://guidance.nice.org.uk/CG22/

National Institute for Health and Clinical Excellence. *Depression (amended): Management of depression in primary and secondary care*. NICE guideline CG23. NICE, London, 2007. http://guidance.nice.org.uk/CG23/

CHAPTER 16

Dementia

Chris Ball

OVERVIEW

- Prevalence of dementia increases with age and affects one in five patients over the age of 80
- Presenting features are: amnesia, apraxia, agnosia, aphasia and associated symptoms (these usually precipitate presentation)
- The history, particularly a collateral history from a carer, is most important in making a diagnosis; cognitive testing with the Mini-Mental State Examination (MMSE) establishes a baseline and is useful in monitoring progress
- Acetylcholinesterase-inhibiting drugs produce an initial improvement in cognition but they do not prevent future decline
- Behavioural problems are the principal reason for referral to specialist services; treatment with antipsychotic drugs is limited by their side effects

Table 16.1 Prevalence of dementia in the UK.

Age (years)	Prevalence
40–65	1 in 1000
65–70	1 in 50
70–80	1 in 20
80+	1 in 5

Box 16.1 **Number of people with dementia in the UK**

England	652,600
Scotland	63,700
Northern Ireland	17,100
Wales	41,800
Total	**775,200**

Estimated by the Alzheimer's Society using population data for 2001

If it were not for dementia there would probably be no older adults' mental health services. Increasing recognition of dementia and the introduction of the first effective treatments for the symptoms of Alzheimer's disease have lead to radical restructuring of many services.

Prevalence

Incidence and prevalence of dementia increases with age (Table 16.1). Above the age of 90 the risk of developing dementia levels off. The principal time of risk for developing the illness is between 70 and 80. It remains the case that dementia is often thought of as an inevitable part of ageing and dismissed as a result. The prevalence of cognitive impairment in non-specialist nursing homes in the UK is of the order of 74% (Box 16.1).

Pathology

Dementia is a syndrome with many underlying causes (Box 16.2).

Box 16.2 **Pathological causes of dementia in those over 70 years of age**

Dementia type	Percentage
Alzheimer type dementia (AD)	50
Lewy body dementia (LBD)	20
Vascular dementia (VD)	10
Mixed AD/VD	10
Other/unknown	10

Presenting features

Symptoms common to the diagnosis of dementia from varying causes may be summarised as the 'five As':
- **Amnesia**, especially for new material, is usually the first problem noted (and often dismissed). The symptom of memory problems has come to dominate to the extent that many dementia services are called 'memory services'. It is argued that this avoids the stigma that comes with the word dementia
- **Apraxia** is manifest as awkwardness in performing tasks. Dressing apraxia is probably the commonest of these problems

ABC of Mental Health, 2nd edition. Edited by T. Davies and T. Craig.
© 2009 Blackwell Publishing, ISBN: 978-0-7279-1639-6.

baseline for, and check on the effectiveness of, treatment. The maximum score on the MMSE is 30: 25–30 is normal, and 20–24 denotes possible mild dementia; 10–20 indicates moderate, and <10 severe, dementia. Care should be taken to ensure a low score is not due to the patient's linguistic or communication difficulties, another illness or disability (e.g. sensory impairment).

Physical examination with particular attention to cardiovascular risk factors and neurological problems should be a routine part of clinical assessment (Box 16.5).

- **Agnosia**. The inability to understand sensory stimuli can make the tasks of everyday living very difficult, and the failure to recognise faces (prosopagnosia) is very distressing to carers
- **Aphasia**. An inability to find words and express needs and feelings leads to frustration on the part of both the sufferer and his or her carers
- **Associated symptoms**. Most commonly, it is the plethora of associated symptoms that brings the person with dementia to the attention of medical services (Box 16.3).

The diagnostic process

There has been increasing recognition that dementia should be diagnosed early in its course (Box 16.4). This has always been the case, but the therapeutic nihilism prior to the introduction of acetylcholinesterase inhibitors (ACIs) was such that this rarely happened.

The most important part of making a diagnosis is the history, particularly a collateral history from an informant, usually a carer. The following questions for informants assist in detecting early dementia:

- Have there been changes in personality?
- Has there been increased forgetfulness or anxiety about forgetting things?
- Have activities or hobbies been given up, and why?
- Has there been confusion or muddle when out of the normal routine?
- Has there been a surprising failure to recognise people (e.g. distant relatives)?
- Has there been any difficulty in speech such as finding words?
- Have the changes been gradual or has there been a sudden worsening?

Formal cognitive testing with a recognised instrument such as the Mini-Mental State Examination (MMSE) or Abbreviated Mental Test Score (AMTS) is useful if indicated by the history, and as a

Giving a diagnosis

Dementia seems to occupy the place that cancer did 10–20 years ago. The diagnosis is often given to the family of the sufferer and not the patient himself or herself. It can be difficult to talk about the diagnosis to the patient with dementia. Careful consideration needs to be given to how to break the diagnosis. A series of questions should be considered before giving a diagnosis:

- When should it be given?
- Who should give it?
- Whom should it be given to?
- Where should it be given?
- How often should it be given?
- What if the diagnosis is not accepted?
- What else might people need at the same time (information) and in the future?

Managing dementia

Increasingly, the diagnostic process takes place in memory clinics established to assess patients with Alzheimer's disease for treatment with ACIs. Memory clinics must also have the capacity to manage those conditions in which the 'obvious' step of drug prescription is not warranted (e.g. vascular dementias), and those in whom the medications are ineffective (Box 16.6).

Acetylcholinesterase inhibitors

After initial controversy about their availability on the NHS, ACIs have moved into mainstream practice. Following a judicial review in 2007, NICE recommended that three ACIs (donepezil, galantamine and rivastigmine) should be used only in the management of patients with Alzheimer's disease of moderate severity (i.e. MMSE score of 10–20 points out of the possible maximum

Box 16.6 **Roles of memory clinics**

- Provide a local focus for people with dementia or suspected dementia
- Access to specialist multidisciplinary assessment
- Systematic cognitive assessment
- Specialist investigations (e.g. CT, MRI)
- Medication prescribing and management
- Psychological (e.g. diagnostic counselling) and social (including financial) interventions
- Education and training
- Carer support
- Contact with non-statutory organisations
- Facilitating pathways into mainstream mental health services

Box 16.7 **NICE guidance on use of acetylcholinesterase inhibitors (ACIs)**

- Alzheimer's disease of moderate severity only (MMSE score 10–20)
- Treatment must be initiated by specialists in the care of patients with dementia
- Carers' views should be sought both before and during treatment
- Treatment should be reviewed every six months using the MMSE, and global, functional and behavioural assessments
- Reviews should be undertaken by an appropriate specialist team
- The drug should be continued only if the patient's MMSE score remains at or above 10 points, and other assessments indicate the drug is having a worthwhile effect

score of 30) (Box 16.7). Memantine may be used only for moderately severe to severe Alzheimer's disease as part of a clinical trial.

Most studies of ACI usage show an improvement in cognition with a return to baseline over 6 months. However, they do not prevent decline, which then parallels the non-treatment group. In clinical practice, between 50% and 60% of people continue medication for longer than 3 months. It is often difficult to decide when the drug should be stopped. Long-term benefits have yet to be clearly demonstrated. It remains questionable if these medications reduce the cost of care, reduce carer burden, delay institutionalisation, or alter the disease process fundamentally.

Referral to mental health services

There are several indications for referring a patient with dementia to mental health services:

- If diagnosis is uncertain
- If certain behavioural and psychological symptoms are present, e.g. aggressive behaviour
- If there are safety concerns, e.g. wandering
- For risk assessment, e.g. if the older person is thought to be at risk of abuse or self-harm
- If there is a need for specialist assessment of dementia, e.g. testamentary capacity or driving
- For treatment with antidementia drugs in accordance with local protocols

- If the patient has complex or multiple problems, e.g. where a patient needs specialist methods of communication due to his or her sensory impairments
- Where there is dual diagnosis, e.g. possible dementia and learning disability, or dementia and other severe mental disorders.

In practice, behavioural disturbance is the principal reason for referral to specialist services

Managing behavioural disturbances in dementia

Whilst some problems emerge directly out of the neurological damage caused by the underlying pathology (e.g. hallucinations in Lewy body dementia), often it is not clear why people with identical degrees of cognitive impairment might present in radically different ways (Figure 16.1). In addition to neurological damage it is important to think about the person who has the illness: what are their life experiences, what are their experiences of illness, and how are they being treated now they have dementia?

Malignant social pathology

Kitwood delineated the role of social processes and procedures in damaging the self-esteem of the dementia sufferer. These set up a self-fulfilling spiral of decline, often resulting in the behavioural disturbances exhibited by the patient (Box 16.8). The major processes are:

- Routines and practices that tend to depersonalise the person with dementia
- Failure to meet the individual patient's needs
- Focus on management, containment and control.

Assessing behavioural disturbance

When a person with dementia presents with behavioural disturbance, a number of questions should be asked before any intervention is commenced:

- What is the 'problem'? (i.e. an operational definition is required)
- To whom is it a problem?
- What is known about the people who are experiencing the problem?
- What is being communicated by the problem?
- How do we find out what is being communicated by the problem?

Box 16.8 **Examples of malignant social pathology**

Accusation	Invalidation
Banishment	Labelling
Disempowerment	Mockery
Disparagement	Objectification
Ignoring	Outpacing
Imposition	Stigma
Infantilisation	Treachery
Intimidation	Withholding

Trying to understand the problem behaviour in this model means that behavioural, psychological and environmental interventions should be considered before medication is used. Lack of trained staff is cited frequently as a reason for not pursuing such interventions: coupled with the demand that 'something must be done', this leads too frequently to the inappropriate and excessive use of medication.

Medication management

If medication is to be considered, the treatment plan must enunciate clearly the likely risks and weigh these against the expected benefits.

- Is it a symptom that will be responsive to drugs?
- Does the symptom warrant drug treatment? And why? (e.g. is it severe and in need of quick resolution?)
- Which medication? (e.g. conventional neuroleptics should not be used in Lewy body disease)
- What are the predictable and potential side effects?
- How long should it be continued? (a review date should be given).

The starting dose of any medication should be low, and dose increased gradually until the 'problem' symptom is controlled adequately or unwanted effects become unacceptable to the patient.

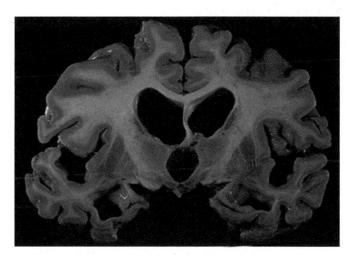

Figure 16.1 Brain of a person with Alzheimer's disease shows gross atrophy but gives few clues about cause of behaviour disturbance in the sufferer.

There is little high-quality evidence of the effectiveness of medication in behavioural symptoms of dementia. The best evidence was for risperidone and olanzapine in the management of aggression, agitation and psychosis. Unfortunately, these drugs were found to increase the risk of stroke in people with dementia approximately threefold. In 2004, the Committee on Safety of Medicines (CSM) recommended that these drugs should no longer be used in these circumstances. For many, this has meant a return to conventional neuroleptics with their complex side effect profiles.

Further information

Alzheimer's Society, http://www.alzheimers.org.uk/

Further reading

Burns A, Howard R, Petit W. *Alzheimer's disease: A medical companion.* Blackwell Science, Oxford, 1995.

Cantley, C (ed.). *A handbook of dementia care.* Open University Press, Buckingham, 2001.

Department of Health. *National Service Framework for Older People.* DH, London, 2001. http://www.dh.gov.uk/en/Publicationsandstatistics/Publications/PublicationsPolicyAndGuidance/DH_4003066

Folstein MF, Folstein SE, McHugh PR. 'Mini-mental state'. A practical method for grading the cognitive state of patients for the clinician. *J Psychiatric Res* 1975; **12**: 189–98.

Kitwood T. *Dementia reconsidered. The person comes first.* Open University Press, Buckingham, 1997.

Macdonald AJD, Carpenter GI, Box O, *et al.* Dementia and use of psychotropic medication in non-elderly mentally infirm nursing homes in South East England. *Age Ageing*, 2002; **31**: 58–64.

Marriott H. *The selfish pig's guide to caring.* Time Warner, London, 2006.

National Institute for Health and Clinical Excellence. *Dementia: Supporting people with dementia and their carers in health and social care.* NICE guideline CG42. NICE, London, 2006. http://guidance.nice.org.uk/CG42/

National Institute for Health and Clinical Excellence. *Donepezil, galantamine, rivastigmine (review) and memantine for the treatment of Alzheimer's disease (amended).* NICE technology appraisal guidance 111 (amended). NICE, London, 2007. www.nice.org.uk/TA111

CHAPTER 17

Mental Health Problems of Children and Adolescents

Emily Simonoff

OVERVIEW

- Psychiatric disorders occur in about 20% of children; their aetiology, development and presentation are greatly influenced by the child's psychosocial environment

- Presence of psychosocial impairment usually defines the threshold for intervention and treatment

- Child psychiatric disorders can be divided into three groups: behavioural disorders, emotional disorders and disorders affecting development

- Most psychotherapies for children require parental participation

- Child and adolescent mental health services should provide rapid access for all children with significant mental health problems and their families

Psychiatric disorders in children and adolescents are common, frequently persistent over time, and likely to cause impairment in psychosocial functioning. Many mental health problems in children and adolescents go undetected for long periods of time because parents, other carers and teachers are unaware of the symptoms, fail to recognise the symptoms as forming part of a psychiatric disorder, or are unaware of the potential role for treatment.

From April 2008, increasing use of the Common Assessment Framework (CAF), especially in schools, should help in identifying a child's difficulties and needs earlier. The CAF facilitates gathering of information from several sources about a child's personal development, the quality of parenting and the influence of wider environmental factors, all of which can provide evidence to support further investigation.

The general practitioner provides an invaluable intermediate step in recognising and disentangling symptoms of emotional and behavioural disorders and providing a conduit for referral to the appropriate services.

ABC of Mental Health, 2nd edition. Edited by T. Davies and T. Craig.
© 2009 Blackwell Publishing, ISBN: 978-0-7279-1639-6.

Risk factors for child mental health problems

The presence of risk factors can alert the GP to probe more carefully for the symptoms of a psychiatric disorder in a child with a non-specific presentation. Important family factors include parental physical and mental disorder and domestic violence. The risk may be mediated through a number of routes: parenting may be suboptimal, children may be expected to take on increased responsibilities including caring for parents, or children may witness severe violence.

Adequate parenting requires the provision of appropriate support and nurturing, the encouragement to develop independence while simultaneously providing adequate supervision, with clear boundaries and contingent reinforcement (praise or punishment) for behaviour. Living in poverty, unsuitable housing, or an unsafe neighbourhood are also risk factors for child psychiatric disorder, although the routes to disorder are not entirely clear. While environmental deprivation and danger may provide one source of risk, these factors may also be associated with other characteristics of parents and family functioning that will not be immediately repaired by a change in family financial or housing circumstances. Nevertheless, negative experiences, both family and externally based, may play an important role in initiating psychiatric symptoms.

With increasing recognition of post-traumatic stress disorder in children, it is important to elicit any significant life events or experiences. Children are surprisingly reluctant to tell their parents about bullying at school or in their peer environment, and more sensitive areas of abuse may be even more difficult to discuss. Environmental triggers frequently play a role, but should be considered especially in children with a relatively sudden onset in the context of previously good functioning. Of course, chronic environmental threat will frequently produce a clinical picture of chronic psychiatric disorder.

Family factors may also play a role in determining the outcome of disorder. Parental recognition of psychiatric symptoms plays a crucial role in determining referral to and attendance at mental health services. This divergence in opinion may stem from several routes. First, the child's behaviour may differ in varying situations, so that reports from school of disruptive and antisocial behaviour may not coincide with parents' perspective from home. Second, the same behaviour may be interpreted in different ways.

Inattentive, fidgety behaviour at school may be seen as normal boisterousness in a less structured context. Third, concepts of the origins of problem behaviour may differ: 'bad' rather than 'disturbed'.

In addition to having different conceptualisations of behaviour, other parental characteristics may interfere with help-seeking. Parents' own illnesses may reduce their capacity to attend appointments for their child and to engage in the cognitive and practical aspects of implementing treatment. The majority of psychotherapies for children require parental participation and may founder if this is not forthcoming. For all these reasons, developing a shared collaborative relationship with parents from the outset is an important component of treatment.

Classification of mental disorders of childhood and adolescence

Psychiatric disorders have been estimated to occur in about 20% of children, but only about half of these experience psychosocial impairment, which is commonly used as the threshold by which to define the need for treatment. 'Psychosocial impairment' refers to a significant effect of symptoms on functioning in one of the areas in which children are expected to perform: relationships with family, peers and other adults; school work and other aspects of school life; and leisure activities.

Child psychiatric disorders can be divided broadly into three groups (Box 17.1): externalising or behavioural disorders, internalising or emotional disorders, and disorders affecting general development. While such a categorisation is helpful, many children presenting with one psychiatric disorder will meet criteria for further psychiatric diagnoses. This comorbidity may complicate the presenting picture and influence treatment options. A comprehensive assessment at the outset is important in gaining a full picture of the nature of the problem, the contributing risk factors and the possible treatment options.

Behavioural disorders

Behavioural disorders are probably most likely to come to the attention of adults because the symptoms are easily observable and have a direct impact on others. Oppositional defiant and conduct disorders refer to a constellation of symptoms in which children display angry, destructive, aggressive and antisocial behaviour. The distinction between the two relates to the spectrum of symptoms with conduct disorder having more severe aggressive and antisocial behaviour and generally occurring in older children and adolescents. The importance of early identification of these two disorders is that appropriate treatment during primary school years has been demonstrated consistently to reduce the disorder. Oppositional defiant and conduct disorders account for roughly half of all referrals to Child and Adolescent Mental Health Services (CAMHS).

The treatment shown to be effective is a specific form of 'parent training' in which parents are taught the principles of contingent behavioural reinforcement (both positive and negative), and given support through therapy in modelling and carrying out these behavioural responses. The fact that parent training is the most effective treatment does not necessarily imply that faulty parenting is the underlying cause of the problem. Although this may be true in a proportion of cases, other child-based and environment-based factors may contribute to the development of oppositional behaviour, which is best treated by appropriate boundaries and contingent behavioural response from parents. There is less systematic research on treatment during adolescence but what is available suggests that parent-based intervention alone may be ineffective (presumably in large part because the social networks of adolescents are so much wider), and multisystems therapy (MST), a more comprehensive and more expensive treatment, is the only intervention shown to lead to significant improvement.

Attention deficit hyperactivity disorder (ADHD) comprises a cluster of symptoms including overactivity, inattention and impulsivity, and affects some 3–5% of the population. In the UK, many practitioners continue to make reference to the more severe form of the disorder, as defined by the International Classification of Diseases, termed 'hyperkinetic disorder'. The latter requires all three symptom areas to be present, and for symptoms to be pervasive across domains of functioning, i.e. home, school and leisure activities. This more severe disorder is present in 1–3% of school-aged children.

Although milder cases of ADHD may show a good response to behavioural intervention, more severe ADHD and hyperkinetic disorder are unlikely to show a good response to behavioural treatment alone, while medication will substantially improve symptoms in up to 90% of children. NICE guidance indicates that the diagnosis and initial treatment of ADHD should be conducted by a child specialist, either a child psychiatrist or community paediatrician with expertise in behavioural disorders. Once a satisfactory medication regimen has been implemented, routine prescribing can be maintained by GPs, with back-up and regular reviews from a child specialist. Many children with ADHD also show elements of

---

Box 17.1 **Main mental disorders of childhood and adolescence**

Behavioural (externalising) disorders
- Oppositional defiant disorder
- Conduct disorder
- Attention deficit hyperactivity disorder (hyperkinetic disorder)

Emotional (internalising) disorders
- Anxiety disorders
  - Separation anxiety
  - Specific phobia
  - Social phobia
  - Agoraphobia
- Depressive disorder
- Obsessive–compulsive disorder
- Eating disorder

Developmental disorders
- Global learning disability
- Specific learning disability
- Pervasive developmental disorder
- Other neuropsychiatric disorders

aggressive and antisocial behaviour and the possibility of ADHD should always be considered in such a presentation, because of the role of a specific treatment approach.

Emotional disorders

Emotional, or internalising, disorders may be less easily recognised by parents, teachers and other adults caring for children, because the symptoms are more subtle and less likely to impinge on adults. Children may not recognise their experiences as symptoms and may not share them with parents or other adults. It is, therefore, particularly important to make specific enquiries of both parent and child to elicit emotional disorders.

Phobias

While specific phobias (dogs, the dark, lifts) are the most common psychiatric disorder of childhood, probably only a third of these cause psychosocial impairment. Nevertheless, most are readily treatable by a behavioural nurse or psychologist using desensitisation and graded exposure to the feared stimulus. Without treatment, symptoms may be persistent. Other phobias, including social phobia, are more likely to cause additional impairment and usually need specialist treatment.

Depression

Depression is uncommon during childhood, affecting less than 1%, but rates increase substantially during adolescence. Although the evidence for pharmacotherapy, both conventional tricyclic antidepressants and selective serotonin reuptake inhibitors (SSRIs), is equivocal, there are now a number of studies demonstrating the benefits of psychological therapy, both cognitive behavioural therapy (CBT) and interpersonal therapy (IPT).

Obsessive–compulsive disorder

Obsessive–compulsive disorder (OCD) in children and adolescents shares its clinical features with the disorder as seen in adulthood, although the nature of the obsessions and compulsions may be different. Children may be more prone to magical thinking and may show simpler thoughts and rituals. Unlike in adults, where the symptoms of OCD are recognised as irrational and foreign, this may not be the case for children. In addition, a proportion of children presenting with symptoms of OCD may have features of a pervasive developmental disorder (PDD) as well. Obsessive–compulsive disorder in children responds to both behavioural treatment and pharmacotherapy (usually with SSRIs).

Eating disorders

The eating disorders anorexia and bulimia nervosa frequently commence during the teenage years, with a minority of cases of anorexia nervosa having onset pre-pubertally. Patients tend to be secretive about their symptoms, so these may have been ongoing for some time before coming to clinical attention. Concern is usually raised by parents, and young people may continue to deny or minimise symptoms. Treatment centres on restoring proper weight and eating habits, either through a family therapy approach, the preferred option if young people are living at home, or individual CBT. Medication may be used to treat comorbid disorders.

Developmental disorders

Level of intelligence is one of the strongest predictors of the presence or absence of child psychiatric disorders, with highly intelligent children being most resilient to psychiatric morbidity in the face of adversity and those with learning disability being at greatest risk. Up to 30–50% of children with a global learning disability also have a psychiatric disorder. In those with severe to profound learning disability, specialist skills within CAMHS are required for both assessment and treatment.

Specific developmental disorders are all associated with an increased rate of psychiatric disorder, including both speech and language disorders, as well as ADHD and other behavioural disorders. Again, a systematic approach to assessment is necessary to identify the entire range of problems and develop a rational treatment plan. Both general and specific learning disabilities can go undetected without a cognitive assessment, performed either by an educational psychologist or the CAMHS team.

Child and Adolescent Mental Health Services (CAMHS)

There has been wide variation across the UK in the availability and type of mental health services for children and adolescents. Recent initiatives, including substantial increases in government funding specifically for CAMHS and the National Service Framework for Children (NSF-Children), should increase the range and uniformity of services. In the future, GPs should expect access to both uniprofessional and multidisciplinary mental health services for children and adolescents. There is at present no overall consensus about the exact way in which services should be organised locally but there is general agreement that CAMHS should be structured to provide rapid and easy access for all children with significant mental health problems and their families. This framework should ordinarily include generic services for the assessment and treatment of common and relatively uncomplicated problems, possibly delivered by a single professional who may work in a CAMHS setting, a GP service, in school or in social services. In addition, multidisciplinary teams should be available to deal with disorders that are rarer, have greater complexity, or require a highly specialised training for their assessment and treatment.

Local services should make their access points clear to GPs and other referrers, including mechanisms for dealing with psychiatric emergencies. An ongoing area of discussion remains the interface between CAMHS, education and social services. Children's Trusts, arising from the UK government's 'Every child matters' strategy, are aimed in part at reducing the debate between services about where responsibility lies. In addition, much of the initial new money for CAMHS has been streamed through education and social services, to provide bridges. However, many Children's Trusts will be virtual rather than real and it is likely that some disagreements will remain. General practitioners have an important role through their Primary Care Trust in directing the development of their local CAMHS in ensuring that the needs of their child patients are met.

Further information

ADDISS (The National Attention Deficit Disorder Information and Support Service), tel. 020 8906 0354, www.addiss.co.uk
ADHD UK Alliance, tel. 020 7608 8760, www.adhdalliance.org.uk
Children's Workforce Development Council, www.cwdcouncil.org.uk
The National Family and Parenting Institute, tel. 020 7424 3460, www.nfpi.org
YoungMinds, www.youngminds.org.uk

Personal accounts of mental health problems

Hughes PJ. *Me and Planet Weirdo*. Chipmunkapublishing, Brentwood, Essex, 2007. www.chipmunka.com
Telfer J. *Christopher's story*. Chipmunkapublishing, Brentwood, Essex, 2006. www.chipmunka.com
Wealthall K. *Little steps*. Chipmunkapublishing, Brentwood, Essex, 2005. www.chipmunka.com

Further reading

Department for Education and Skills. *A quick guide to common assessment.* http://www.dfes.gov.uk/commoncore/docs/CAFQuickGuide.doc
Department for Education and Skills. *Every child matters: Change for children.* DfES, London, 2004. Available from the Children's Workforce Development Council, http://www.cwdcouncil.org.uk/resources/everychildmatters.asp
Department of Health. *National Service Framework for Children, Young People and Maternity Services. Core standards.* DH, London, 2004. http://www.dh.gov.uk/en/Publicationsandstatistics/Publications/PublicationsPolicyAndGuidance/DH_4089099
National Institute for Health and Clinical Excellence. *Depression in children and young people: Identification and management in primary, community and secondary care.* NICE guideline CG28. NICE, London, 2005. http://guidance.nice.org.uk/CG28/
National Institute for Health and Clinical Excellence. *Methylphenidate, atomoxetine and dexamfetamine for attention deficit hyperactivity disorder (ADHD) in children and adolescents. Review of technology appraisal 13.* Technology appraisal 98. NICE, London, 2006. http://guidance.nice.org.uk/TA98/
National Institute for Health and Clinical Excellence. *Attention deficit hyperactivity disorder. Diagnosis and management of ADHD in children, young people and adults.* National clinical practice guideline 72. NICE, London, 2008. http://www.nice.org.uk/nicemedia/pdf/CG72FullGuideline.pdf

CHAPTER 18

Mental Health Problems in People with Intellectual Disability

Nick Bouras and Geraldine Holt

OVERVIEW

- Mental health problems are common in the 2–3% of people with intellectual disability, and may present with challenging behaviours or family dysfunction

- Mental disorders result from complex interactions between biological (e.g. brain damage, epilepsy, sensory impairments) and psychosocial (e.g. abuse, low self-esteem, limited social support, social exclusion) factors

- A full range of psychiatric disorders may present, but people with profound intellectual disability may be unable to communicate their symptoms; clinicians may have to detect signs, such as changes in behaviour, to make a diagnosis

- Treatment options for mental disorders in people with intellectual disability are similar to those for other patients, including pharmacotherapy (using low doses to avoid side effects) and psychosocial interventions

---

Intellectual disability (ID) (Box 18.1) affects approximately 2–3% of people in developed countries and may restrict social, vocational, recreational and educational opportunities. Mental health problems are common in people with ID and may have critical consequences. They may be associated with challenging behaviours, major restrictions in family activities, and increased levels of parental mental illness and sibling dysfunction. They are also a major cause of failure of community residential placements and add major cost to care.

Mental health problems in people with ID are likely to be due to complex interactions between biological and psychosocial factors (Box 18.2). Biological factors include brain damage, epilepsy, sensory impairments, physical illnesses and disabilities, and genetic conditions. Psychosocial factors include rejection, abuse, separations, losses, sexual vulnerability, low self-esteem, limited social and community networks, and social exclusion.

Behavioural phenotypes

Within each syndrome there is a degree of variability. Given that behavioural phenotypes involve probability statements, not

---

Box 18.1 **Definition of intellectual disability**

The term intellectual disability (ID) is equivalent to the International Classification of Diseases rubric mental retardation (ICD 10, F70-73), and to 'learning disability' as used in the UK

- A condition arising during the developmental period (in practice usually taken to mean before 18 years) resulting in the arrested or incomplete development of the mind
- Characterised by an overall level of intellectual functioning that is significantly lower than the general population in terms of cognitive abilities, language, motor and social abilities
- A typical IQ would be less than 70

Box 18.2 **Mental health problems in people with intellectual disability**

- Are common (e.g. prevalence of schizophrenia is about 3%; cf. <1% in general adult population)
- Have significant consequences for the patient, his or her family and others who support them
- May lead to placement breakdown
- Are associated with biological, psychological and social vulnerability factors

---

everyone with a given syndrome will exhibit that syndrome's characteristic behaviours. For example, studies have found that patients with Down syndrome (both children and adults) are more likely to show specific deficits in grammar, expressive language and articulation, than other people with ID, but do not do so invariably. Similarly, those with fragile X syndrome or with Williams syndrome are more likely to be hyperactive, and those with Prader–Willi syndrome to have obsessions and compulsions. Sometimes a particular behaviour is characteristic of, although not necessarily unique to, a particular genetic aetiology, for example: hyperphagia in Prader–Willi syndrome; extreme self-mutilation in Lesch–Nyhan syndrome; schizophrenia in adults with velocardiofacial syndrome; the insertion of foreign objects into bodily orifices (along with the 'self-hugging') in Smith Magenis syndrome.

ABC of Mental Health, 2nd edition. Edited by T. Davies and T. Craig.
© 2009 Blackwell Publishing, ISBN: 978-0-7279-1639-6.

Autism and related disorders

Diagnosing mental illness in people on the autistic spectrum (communication impairments, associated ID) poses several problems. Diagnostic overshadowing, the tendency to report only positive associations, and sampling bias, are among reasons that is it difficult to interpret research findings in this area.

Autism and related disorders, such as Asperger syndrome, may be associated with ID and comorbid mental health problems, in particular depression. However, patients with autism are not at increased risk of schizophrenia.

Relationship between psychiatric disorders and challenging behaviour

The causes of challenging behaviour (Box 18.3) are multifactorial and include physical health problems, epilepsy, behavioural phenotypes, and communication and sensory difficulties. Some challenging behaviours may be developmentally appropriate in a patient with more severe ID. They may be caused or exacerbated by a coexisting psychiatric disorder, and this might provide the motivational basis for challenging behaviour. For example, a patient who is depressed might not want to do much, and might behave in a challenging manner if people try to encourage him or her to engage in activities. This may set up a pattern whereby the patient learns to behave in this way to avoid unwanted activities, and those who provide support learn to avoid confrontation by not encouraging activities. Challenging behaviours may be the atypical presentation of mental illness, e.g. self-injurious behaviours (SIB) may be the manifestation of obsessive–compulsive disorder in someone with severe ID.

Assessment and diagnosis

Assessment of mental health problems (Box 18.4) of people with ID presents several challenges.

Patients are less likely to seek help themselves

Most referrals are initiated by distressed carers, rather than distressed patients. It is necessary to ensure that a patient with ID understands why he or she has been referred to a mental health professional, and to understand and respect their views on whether they want to be seen. Clinicians also need to consider the reasons why an assessment has been requested. It is easy for staff to attribute behaviours such as aggression to the internal state of the patient, when it may be the environment, or behaviour of staff or others that is causing the patient to act in a particular way. However, the opposite can occur and patients may not be referred to mental health services as staff believe that behaviour is due to external influences: this is known as behavioural overshadowing. Staff attitudes and their own experiences of mental health services may well influence the assessment of the patient.

Process of the mental health assessment may need to be adapted

Patients may have a reduced attention span and be distractible (so several short assessment sessions in a quiet environment may be needed). Patients may be suggestible and acquiescent, telling clinicians what they believe they want to hear. They may pretend to understand what is being said, so as not to appear incompetent (ask the same question in different ways, use simple words and anchoring events). Communication impairments may inhibit the patient's ability to describe his or her feelings and experiences (communication aids such as pictures or symbols may be helpful, information from people who know the patient may be vital).

Significance of symptoms and signs may be altered

Changes in the patient's state of mind and his or her behaviours are particularly important pointers to the possibility of a mental illness. The assessor needs to be aware that staff who support people with ID often lack experience and knowledge of mental health. Also, staff turnover may result in an incomplete knowledge of the patient's history and current situation. The patient's altered trajectory of development and their usual level of functioning and behaviours should be taken into account (someone may appear to talk in response to auditory hallucinations, but may instead be talking to his or her longstanding imaginary friend). People with autism may have monotone speech, echolalia and neologisms (which may be misinterpreted as suggestive of mental illness) and have particular difficulties in describing their feelings.

Assessment process should be multidisciplinary

Mental health problems in patients with ID are frequently caused and maintained by multiple factors. A multidisciplinary approach enables a comprehensive assessment including review of existing records, interviews with the patient, family members and support staff, physical examination, functional behavioural analysis and direct observations, and specialist assessments (e.g. communication skills). This approach attempts to explain the possible inter-relationship between biological, psychological, social and environmental factors in causing and maintaining the patient's difficulties.

Application of standardised diagnostic criteria for psychiatric disorders is problematic in people with ID

People with ID have been excluded from trials of standardised diagnostic criteria raising the question of whether the results apply to this population. The Diagnostic Criteria for psychiatric disorders for use with adults with Learning Disabilities (DC-LD) uses modified versions of ICD-10 diagnostic criteria for non-affective psychoses, attention deficit hyperactivity disorder (ADHD), anxiety disorders, depressive disorders and eating disorders. It gives a classification of problem behaviours, and applies the diagnostic criteria to behavioural phenotypes. The use of structured and semi-structured interviews, e.g. the Psychiatric Assessment Schedule for Adults with Developmental Disability (PAS-ADD), has significantly increased the reliability of the diagnostic process in psychiatry.

Functional assessment and analysis may be indicated

This may be needed to identify variables that affect the occurrence of behaviours, and includes techniques of indirect, descriptive and analogue assessments. This model has been successful in providing explanations of, and treatment for, challenging behaviours in people with ID including self-injury, aggression and a wide range of other maladaptive behaviours. A variety of psychiatric disorders in people with ID have been successfully analysed and treated using information from functional analysis including mood and anxiety disorders.

Psychiatric disorders

People with ID can experience the full range of psychiatric disorders; however, the presentation may vary (Box 18.5). People with mild ID generally have a similar presentation to those without ID. With the right support and approach to interviewing, usually they can describe symptoms such as hallucinations, delusions and feelings associated with altered mood. But for people with severe and profound ID and communication difficulties, it is extremely difficult to elicit descriptions of their internal world, and the clinician may have to rely on signs, such as changes in behaviour, rather than symptoms in making a diagnosis.

Box 18.5 **Psychiatric disorders**

Schizophrenia
- Prevalence around 3%
- Diagnosis becomes increasingly difficult in more severe ID, and rests on behavioural signs rather than symptoms
- Catatonic and paranoid symptoms are more frequently seen in severe ID
- A trial of treatment is indicated where behavioural signs suggest that psychotic symptoms are present

Mood disorders
- Prevalence estimated to be 1.3–4.4%; Down syndrome increases the risk
- Depression in patients with severe ID may present with biological features and atypical signs

Anxiety disorders
- Prevalence of anxiety disorders is thought to be higher than in the general population
- Anxiety may present with aggression and self-harm
- Obsessive–compulsive disorders may present with atypical features (compulsions, self-injurious behaviours, stereotypies)
- Phobias may be compatible with the patient's developmental level
- Possibility of physical or sexual abuse must be considered

Dementia
- Dementia is very common (10–30%)
- Patients with Down syndrome have a greater risk of developing Alzheimer's disease

Eating disorders
- Prevalence 1–19% of those living in the community; 3–42% of those living in institutions
- Highest rates found in those with more severe ID

Personality disorder
- Prevalence ranges from 22% to 25% of those with mild to moderate ID
- Diagnosis should not be made in patients with severe ID, nor before the patient is over 21 years

---

Schizophrenia

The estimated prevalence of schizophrenia in people with ID is around 3%, with the highest rate in those with mild and borderline intellectual disability. Those with indicators for organic conditions (such as hearing impairment, low birth weight, prematurity and obstetric complications) and a positive family history for schizophrenia are at increased risk.

In people with mild ID and good verbal skills the presentation is similar to those without ID. In people with moderate ID and limited language abilities diagnosis is more dependent on the longitudinal history with a decline in functioning and changes in behaviour suggestive of underlying psychotic illness. Catatonia and paranoid symptoms are more readily identifiable in this group. For those with severe ID it is virtually impossible to diagnose schizophrenia with confidence due to limitations in communication. Where a patient does not meet the diagnostic criteria for schizophrenia, but from the history and behavioural observation it is hypothesised that psychotic symptoms are present, a working diagnosis might be made that is tested through clinical outcomes of treatment.

Mood disorders

Prevalence of depressive disorders in people with ID is estimated to be 1.3–4.4%. People with Down syndrome may be particularly at risk. The clinical features vary with the level of disability. People with mild ID present similarly to the general population, whereas those with severe ID may present with biological features, including changes in appetite and sleep, together with atypical signs such as screaming, aggression, self-injurious behaviour, reduced communication and irritable mood. Some diagnostic criteria are developmentally dependent and cannot easily be assessed in patients with limited conceptual and language skills (e.g. feelings of worthlessness or guilt, suicidal ideation).

Cyclical changes in affect (i.e. the outward expression of inner mood states) and activity level may be suggestive of recurrent affective illness. A daily record of mood and activity level may be useful in clarifying a diagnosis. Rapid cycling bipolar affective disorder (more than four episodes a year) appears to be more prevalent in those with an ID.

Anxiety disorders

The reported prevalence of anxiety disorders varies dramatically in people with ID. It is thought to be higher than in the general population, possibly because of the increased likelihood of physical illness, trauma and abuse. People with Down syndrome are more prone to anxiety and obsessive–compulsive disorder (OCD) following traumatic events. Anxiety disorders reported in people with ID include generalised anxiety disorder, phobias and panic attacks, OCD and post-traumatic stress disorder (PTSD). In addition to the typical signs and symptoms of anxiety, people with ID may show aggressive and self-injurous behaviours.

It may be challenging to diagnose obsessions in people with ID if they have difficulty describing their thoughts. However, compulsions are readily observable, as is the mounting anxiety or tension when a compulsion is prevented or interrupted. Compulsive behaviours have reported frequencies of 3.5% in those with mild to moderate ID. Compulsions, self-injurious behaviours and stereotypies may be atypical presentations of OCDs.

Phobias in adults with ID may be compatible with the patient's developmental level. Common fears include fear of the dark, dogs, dentists or blood. Communication impairments make it challenging to explain or dismiss fears when they arise. In addition, over protection from caregivers can lead to learned dependence and avoidance of feared stimuli.

People with ID are particularly vulnerable to physical and sexual abuse. Their reactions may be similar to those without ID, and PTSD symptoms are common. They may be unable to relate the details of the abusive event. It is important for clinicians to be alert to the possibility of abuse.

Dementia

Dementia is more prevalent (10–30%) in those with ID, especially people with Down syndrome who are at particular risk of developing Alzheimer's disease. Global deterioration in functioning is seen.

Diagnosis may be delayed because initial signs and symptoms such as forgetfulness and confusion may be misinterpreted as part of the patient's ID, or not be evident because of the support the patient receives. Treatable conditions that may present similarly or coexist, such as thyroid disorder, hearing or visual impairment and depression, should be excluded.

Eating disorders

The prevalence of eating disorders in adults with ID is estimated to be between 1% and 19% of those living in the community and 3% and 42% of those living in institutions. Higher rates occur in those with more severe ID. Eating disorders include pica, rumination and regurgitation, psychogenic vomiting, food faddiness or refusal and psychogenic loss of appetite, binge eating disorders and anorexia nervosa. They may be associated with an additional psychiatric disorder, and with physical and social comorbidity.

Personality disorder

There has been a slow but steady flow of research on personality disorder (PD) in people with ID. It is a diagnosis that is usually confined to those with mild to moderate ID. Communication difficulties, lack of understanding of the laws and mores of society, and profound developmental delay make the diagnosis inappropriate in those with more severe ID. The diagnosis is not considered clinically appropriate until the patient is over 21 years, due to the slower rate of development of personality characteristics.

Treatment methods

Therapeutic interventions for people with ID and mental health problems are similar for those without ID, including pharmacotherapy and psychosocial interventions (Box 18.6). As with assessments, interventions are often multidisciplinary, aiming to address the specific needs of the patient within their social network. Some interventions are targeted at the 'here and now', to achieve

---

Box 18.6 Treatment methods

Interventions are usually multidisciplinary and aim to:
- Relieve symptoms
- Resolve the illness
- Prevent relapse
- Minimise disability

Pharmacotherapy
- Unwanted effects are common
- Start with low doses of medication; review frequently

Psychological treatment
- Behaviour therapy effective
- Growing evidence of effectiveness of cognitive behavioural and other psychotherapies

Social intervention
- Social and interpersonal needs
- Physical environment
- Family support
- Training for support staff

symptom relief (short-term use of anxiolytics to reduce anxiety) and resolution (treatment of coexisting physical problems, antidepressants to treat depression). Others are aimed at reducing the likelihood of relapse and minimising disability (improving communication skills, cognitive behavioural therapy). Where interventions involve several agencies they should be coordinated using the Care Programme Approach. Staff training and service systems are important considerations in providing environments that enable mental health.

Pharmacotherapy

Pharmacotherapy has been used successfully to treat psychiatric disorders in people with ID. It should be used cautiously as unwanted effects are more common, including paradoxical and toxic reactions. It is advisable to start with low doses of medication, reviewing progress at regular, frequent intervals. Often people with ID will respond to lower doses of drugs than people without ID. Atypical and typical antipsychotics have been used in the management of challenging behaviour as an adjunct to psychological interventions.

Psychosocial interventions

Psychological interventions include behavioural therapy, cognitive behavioural therapy, and other psychotherapies. Behaviour therapy can be very effective. The evidence base for cognitive behavioural therapy and other psychotherapies is relatively weak, although there is beginning to develop sufficient conceptual and outcome data to suggest that such interventions should be made routinely available to people with ID and mental health problems.

Environmental and social triggers may be important in the development and maintenance of challenging behaviour and psychiatric disorders. People with autistic spectrum disorders are particularly sensitive to change. Careful planning for inevitable changes may reduce the patient's distress and avoid mental illness. A careful review of living conditions, daily activities, changes in routines and relationships, and staff and family carers' responses to the patient's behaviour, is necessary to understand the context of the patient's distress. Interventions to address a patient's social (access to appropriate activities, individualised support packages, communication training for support staff) and physical (aids and adaptations) environment may transform a patient's quality of life.

Service models

Services for people with ID and mental health problems take various forms. They include provision from mainstream mental health

---

Box 18.7 **Service models**

- Services take various forms
- A specialist service is likely to be necessary for many patients
- The patient, his or her family, carers and other supporters should be involved in development of the care plan

---

services, from specialist mental health services and from a generic ID service with several functions (skill development, needs assessment and social support) including mental health care. There is emerging evidence that some form of specialist service is necessary for this patient group. Specialist ID services have always stressed the importance of the social environment for the quality of lives of people with intellectual disabilities. Therapeutic interventions should be consistent with this. The involvement of the patient with ID, his or her family, and other supporters (if the patient with ID wishes) in the development of the care plan will increase the likelihood that interventions will be appropriate and successful (Box 18.7).

Personal account of mental health problems

Telfer J. *Christopher's story*. Chipmunkapublishing, Brentwood, Essex, 2006. www.chipmunka.com

Further reading

Bouras N, Holt G (eds). *Psychiatric and behavioural disorders in intellectual and developmental disabilities*, 2nd edn. Cambridge University Press, Cambridge, 2007.

Deb S, Matthews T, Holt G, Bouras N. *Practice guidelines for assessment and diagnosis of mental health problems in adults with intellectual disability*. Pavilion Publishing, Brighton, 2001.

Fraser W, Kerr M (eds). *Seminars in the psychiatry of learning disabilities*. Gaskell, London, 2003.

Holt G, Gratsa A, Bouras N, Joyce T, Spiller J, Hardy S. *Guide to mental health for families and carers of people with intellectual disabilities*. Jessica Kingsley Publishers, London, 2004.

Royal College of Psychiatrists. *DC-LD: Diagnostic criteria for psychiatric disorders for use with adults with learning disabilities/mental retardation*. Occasional Paper OP48. RCPsych, London, 2001.

Xenitidis K, Slade M, Thornicroft G, Bouras N. *CANDID: Camberwell assessment of need for adults with developmental and intellectual disabilities*. Gaskell, London, 2003.

CHAPTER 19

Mental Health in a Multiethnic Society

Simon Dein

OVERVIEW

- Culture includes the rules that people use to interpret their world and to act purposefully within it; culture determines what is seen as normal and abnormal, and how distress may be expressed

- Certain behaviours, sanctioned in one society, may be regarded as evidence of mental disorder in another

- Presentation of mental disorder (e.g. schizophrenia, depression) may be modified by cultural factors; and some disorders are 'culture bound' or specific to a particular society or region

- Treatment should take account of the patient's culture and explanatory model of illness

- Many members of ethnic minority groups have experienced racism and this will modify their view of healthcare services, and their acceptance of treatment

Box 19.1 **Depression may present with somatic symptoms**

Mr K, a 52-year-old married man from Delhi, had lived in Britain for over 20 years. He presented to his general practitioner with a two-month history of lethargy, weakness and aching joints. He was subjected to several physical investigations, but no abnormality was detected. When he was interviewed by a Hindi-speaking doctor he admitted to low mood, poor appetite and anhedonia. A diagnosis of depressive disorder was made and he responded well to conventional antidepressant drugs.

According to UK census data, ethnic minorities comprise just over 4.6 million people or about 8% of the British population. Of these, the largest groups are Asian (4%) and black (mainly African or Caribbean, 2%); the remaining 2% arise from a wide range of backgrounds. Their geographical distribution is highly uneven, with most people of black or Asian ethnicity living in greater London, the West Midlands, and other metropolitan counties, whereas recent immigrants from eastern European countries are more evenly dispersed.

The proportion of people from ethnic minorities has increased by about 50% in 10 years, and doctors in Britain increasingly encounter patients whose values and beliefs differ substantially from their own. Without a knowledge of other cultural beliefs and practices, doctors can easily fall prey to errors of diagnosis, resulting in inappropriate management and poor compliance. For example, a delusion is a false belief not amenable to reason and incongruent with a person's cultural and religious beliefs: diagnosing someone as deluded must take into account cultural and religious factors.

Culture refers to the categories, plans and rules that people use to interpret their world and to act purposefully within it. These rules are learned in childhood while growing up in society. Cultural factors relate to mental illness in several ways. In the first instance, culture determines what is seen as normal and abnormal within a given society (Box 19.1).

Normal and abnormal behaviour

Definitions of what constitutes normal and abnormal behaviour vary widely from culture to culture and, within any given group, are dependent on demographic factors such as age and sex, social class and occupation. Behaviours that may be perceived as abnormal at one time may be regarded as normal at other times, such as during carnivals. At these times it is culturally acceptable for men to dress as women or animals.

However, it seems that there is no culture in which men and women remain oblivious to erratic, disturbed, threatening or bizarre behaviour in their midst. This is the more so when such behaviours occur without apparent reason. In some cultures these behaviours may be seen as bad, meriting punishment, whereas in others they may be seen as signs of illness requiring treatment.

Idioms of distress

British doctors may encounter behaviours that in other societies are acceptable, at least sometimes, but that could be interpreted as signs of mental illness: witchcraft and possession states are good examples of this. In many parts of the world these are culturally sanctioned ways of accounting for misfortune or expressing distress and are socially acceptable as such.

ABC of Mental Health, 2nd edition. Edited by T. Davies and T. Craig.
© 2009 Blackwell Publishing, ISBN: 978-0-7279-1639-6.

Obeah is a form of witchcraft containing elements of Christianity, animism, folk medicine and personal malevolence

Obeah

A prevalent belief among immigrants from rural (and sometimes urban) communities of Africa and Asia is that it is possible to influence the health or well-being of another person by action at a distance. Culturally sanctioned ways of dealing with this often involve resorting to traditional healers or the use of countermagic. Among African-Caribbean people in Britain a belief in obeah is common, and various countermeasures are employed.

A doctor presented with someone claiming to have been bewitched may misdiagnose a paranoid disorder and treat the patient with antipsychotic drugs (Box 19.2). Discussion with the family might suggest that involving a traditional healer would be more appropriate and, in the absence of a suitable healer, a Christian priest might be acceptable as many believers in witchcraft also adhere to Christianity.

Possession

This means the takeover of a person's mind and body by an external force such as a spirit or ancestor. The force controls the patient's thoughts and actions and deprives him or her of responsibility for these actions. In many parts of the world people freely admit to being possessed and to having spirits speak and act through them. Anthropologists point out that this mode of expression is deployed by disadvantaged members of a group to gain otherwise unattainable ends. The possessed person seems to be in a trance-like state and may perform actions that are totally out of character.

This state may be misdiagnosed as schizophrenia and treated as such. However, a more satisfactory outcome is likely if an exorcism is performed by the religious authorities, whereas the doctor should pay attention to the interpersonal problems in the patient's family that are likely to have been the precipitants (Box 19.3).

Explanations of mental illness

Each culture provides its members with ways of explaining mental illness, attempting to answer questions about why, and under what circumstances, someone becomes mentally ill. In the West,

emphasis is placed on psychological factors, life events and the effects of stress, but in many parts of the developing world explanations of mental illness take into account wider social and religious factors. These include spirit possession, witchcraft, the breaking of religious taboos, divine retribution and the capture of the soul by a spirit. Thus, these factors may need to be considered if treatment is to be accepted. For example, taking tablets may not make sense to a patient who perceives his or her problems to lie in some religious misdemeanour.

Prognosis of schizophrenia is better in developing societies than in Western ones, and this may relate to support from families who share the patient's beliefs

Presentation of mental illness

Evidence from studies by transcultural psychiatrists and psychologists indicates that the major mental disorders, schizophrenia and depressive illness, occur worldwide.

Schizophrenia

Although the form of the disorder remains constant, culture determines the subjective elements (content) of the illness and the way that it is expressed. Delusions and hallucinations draw on the symbols and images of the patient's cultural milieu. For example, in the West, delusions often relate to technology (such as electricity being put into the brain, or being controlled by a computer), whereas in Africa and India it is more common for delusions to have a religious basis (involving being taken over or harmed by gods or spirits).

Depression

Among people from the Far East and from lower socioeconomic groups in Western cultures, depressive illness may present primarily as physical symptoms (somatisation). Patients from such backgrounds might complain of lethargy and joint pains rather than low mood. Failure to recognise the underlying depression may result in patients being subjected to unnecessary physical investigations, prolonging the symptoms and reinforcing beliefs in their physical nature. Such symptoms are likely to respond to conventional antidepressant treatments.

Box 19.4 **Culture-bound syndromes**

Syndromes of behaviours or beliefs that are specific to certain cultures and reflect core cultural themes
- **Amok:** spree of sudden violent attacks on people, animals or property affecting men in Malaysia
- **Evil eye:** belief among Latin Americans that illness is caused by the stare of a jealous person
- **Jiryan or dhat:** belief amongst men from the Indian subcontinent about leakage of sperm into the urine
- **Koro:** belief that the penis is shrinking into the abdomen
- **Latah:** syndrome of increased suggestibility and imitative behaviour found in South East Asia
- **Susto:** belief in the loss of the soul in Latin America

Culture-bound syndromes

These are culturally determined abnormal behaviour patterns that are specific to a particular culture or geographical region (Box 19.4). The behaviours express core cultural themes and have a wide range of symbolic meanings – social, moral and psychological. It is debatable how these disorders relate to conventional Western categories of mental illness. However, disorders recognised in the West such as anorexia nervosa, agoraphobia and parasuicide may also be regarded as culture-bound syndromes expressing notions of the role of women in developed societies.

Psychosexual disorders

The prevalence of psychosexual disorders among ethnic minorities in Britain is unknown, but it seems likely that most of these disorders are treated by indigenous healers. A common complaint by men from the Indian subcontinent is that sperm is leaking from the body into the urine. This complaint – called jiryan in Pakistan and dhat in India – may be prompted by anxiety over sexual potency or guilt about masturbation, and it may be compounded by cloudiness of the urine secondary to infection. It may also be used to explain various other problems due to organic disease or feelings of depression. It is important to recognise that this widely held belief is not a delusion.

Religion and mental health

Being religious may enhance mental health. There is evidence that intrinsic religiosity, being religious for its own sake rather than for the social benefit it brings, enhances a sense of well-being and can protect against the effect of negative life events. Religion may be protective on account of the cognitive reappraisals it provides and the perceived support of God and of a religious community. Religious professionals such as chaplains may be valuable in making sense of clinical presentations where there is doubt about the religious nature of a patient's beliefs or behaviours.

Migration and mental disorder

Most studies of psychiatric disorder among immigrants to Britain are based on hospital admission records. West Indian immigrants have higher admission rates for schizophrenia than people born in Britain, although there has been concern that this may be accounted for in part by overdiagnosis of schizophrenia in this group. Similarly, the rate of schizophrenia in immigrants from West Africa aged 25–35 has been estimated at nearly 30 times that of the native British population. Whereas about 8% of white patients in psychiatric hospitals are detained under the Mental Health Act, the figure for black patients is about 25%. Men from Northern Ireland are more likely to be admitted with a diagnosis of alcoholism than native British men.

Of course, these statistics have major pitfalls and may not reflect the true prevalence of the disorders in these populations. Factors such as stigmatisation and racism are likely to account for some of the differences in admission rates.

Racial or ethnic discrimination show strong associations with common mental disorders

Two theories have been proposed to account for the purported high prevalence of mental disorder among immigrants. The first is that people who are mentally ill are the ones most likely to emigrate; the second is that the stress of migration results in mental breakdown. There seems to be no single explanation for the differing rates of mental illness that is applicable to all minority or ethnic groups. Without doubt, factors such as dislocation from the native community, rejection by the host community and difficulties in adapting to the cultural norms of the host society, are perceived as intensely stressful and may contribute to mental breakdown in some vulnerable individuals.

Family structure

Norms of family structure amongst immigrants may differ from those of the host country. Asian immigrants to Britain may have extended families, in which couples and their children may live under one roof with grandparents, aunts, uncles and nieces (Box 19.5). Concepts of respect and disrespect, loyalty, independence, position of elders, and obligations to the family and to the wider community, all vary between different ethnic groups. Conflicts arising between family members reflect this complexity.

Box 19.5 **Reactions to stress may present with unexplained physical symptoms**

Mrs B, a 23-year-old newly married woman, was living in her mother-in-law's home while her husband visited his family in Pakistan. She collapsed while making tea for her mother-in-law, and was taken to the local accident and emergency department by ambulance. On examination, there was total loss of power and sensation in the legs but no physical basis was detected. She confided in the interpreter that she missed her husband and was being treated 'like a slave' by his family while he was away. She was empowered to speak to her husband by phone, and he mediated with his parents. Mrs B was discharged home with no residual symptoms.

For example, the marriages of many Indian and Pakistani adults now resident in Britain were arranged for them by their parents. Often, one partner arrived from the home country just before the marriage ceremony while the other had been brought up in Britain. Such partners are likely to hold very different value systems, which, together with the obligation to honour their families' expectations, may place their marriage under considerable strain and lead to marital breakdown.

> Marital and family therapy for ethnic minorities must take into account cultural aspects of family structure or risk creating other problems.
>
> A family therapist's encouragement to a teenage daughter to strive for self-fulfilment may be in direct conflict with her father's views of the authority of the male head of the family and his notion of good conduct

Cultural aspects of treatment

The first step in treating patients from ethnic minority groups is, as with all patients, to decide if a problem exists and, if it does, to clarify its nature and degree. General principles of this process apply to all patients, but to these should be added a knowledge of the culture from which a patient derives. It is important to remember that, for many people from ethnic minorities, their everyday experience of racism is a major factor shaping their presentation and use of health services.

It is vital to find out how a patient seems to members of his or her own culture, and a doctor is likely to benefit from enlisting the help of the patient's family and close friends. Other useful, and often important, informants include religious officials and traditional healers, together with an interpreter when there are linguistic problems. It is, of course, important to be aware that an interpreter (especially if a member of the patient's family) may have a vested interest in presenting the patient as mad if the patient has broken a taboo, has been sexually promiscuous or is resisting family pressures.

It may be decided that a mental health problem does not exist and that the 'patient' is exhibiting culturally appropriate behaviour. In this case, a traditional healer may be more relevant than a general practitioner or psychiatrist. Traditional healers are better at treating certain problems than Western practitioners. For example, hakims (Moslem) and vaids (Hindu) may be better at dealing with psychosexual problems in their community than conventional psychosexual therapists.

When a mental disorder is recognised and it is appropriate to apply Western treatments such as drugs or electroconvulsive therapy, it is still important to elicit the patient's own explanatory model of the illness and attempt to explain the treatment in these terms. This will enhance the patient's trust in the doctor and improve compliance.

Other factors affecting treatment

More work is needed on the different response to psychotropic drugs among different ethnic groups. It seems that South Asian

Box 19.6 **Making mental health services more accessible for ethnic minorities**

Patients
- To be treated with respect
- To be interviewed by staff with relevant language skills, or accompanied by an interpreter
- To be encouraged to explain their views, and to have the views of the doctor explained to them

Doctors and other staff
- To understand issues of racism and stigma in relation to the mental health of ethnic minority groups
- To be aware of, and be instructed in, the cultural norms and religious beliefs of the main ethnic groups consulting them
- To elicit and attempt to understand the explanatory models of illness used by their patients, and to consider the value of traditional healing methods

Ethnic minority groups
- To be provided with information about Western concepts of mental illness and its treatments
- To be consulted and involved in developing services
- To be encouraged to join patient support and advocacy groups

patients show higher plasma concentrations of antidepressants than do white patients given a similar dose. These patients may be more sensitive to side effects and respond to lower doses.

Transcultural psychiatrists have found that management of mental illness in developing countries must take into account not only the patient but also the wider kinship group of which the patient is a member. Treatment aims to resolve tensions among family members that may have been causally related to the patient's illness. Psychiatric management of disorders among ethnic minorities in Britain must also take account of these factors.

Intercultural therapy

Several centres have been established in Britain to provide psychotherapy to ethnic minority groups (Box 19.6). Among the best known is the Nafsiyat Intercultural Therapy Centre in north London. It is funded jointly by the local authority and the health service and offers formal psychotherapy to members of ethnic minority groups, taking account of racial and cultural components in mental disorder. It is involved in organising training courses and seminars in intercultural therapy and in conducting research into the efficacy of treatment.

Further information

Details of programmes for ethnic minorities supported by the Care Services Improvement Partnership (CSIP) are available from http://www.csip.org.uk
African-Caribbean Mental Health Association (020 7737 3603)
Chinese Mental Health Association, http://www.cmha.org.uk
Fanon Care, http://www.southsidepartnership.org.uk/txt/text3.html
Jewish Association for the Mentally Ill, http://www.jamiuk.org
Nafsiyat Intercultural Therapy Centre, http://www.nafsiyat.org.uk
Vietnamese Mental Health Services, http://www.vmhs.org.uk

Personal account of mental health problems

Samuel A. *My longest journey*. Chipmunkapublishing, Brentwood, Essex, 2006. www.chipmunka.com

Further reading

Bhugra D, Bhui K (eds). *Textbook of cultural psychiatry*. Cambridge University Press, Cambridge, 2007.

Bhui K, McKenzie K, Gill P. Delivering mental health services for a diverse society. *BMJ* 2004; **329**: 363–4.

Bhui K, Stansfeld S, McKenzie K, *et al.* Racial/ethnic discrimination and common mental disorders among workers: findings from the EMPIRIC study of ethnic minority groups in the United Kingdom. *Am J Publ Health* 2005; **95**: 496–501.

Chakraborty A, McKenzie K. Does racial discrimination cause mental illness? *Br J Psych* 2002, **180**: 475–7.

Littlewood R, Lipsedge R. *Aliens and alienists. Ethnic minorities and mental health*. Routledge, London, 1997.

Marwaha S, Livingston G. Stigma, racism or choice. Why do depressed ethnic elders avoid psychiatrists? *J Affective Dis* 2002; **72**: 257–65.

Sheikh A, Gatrad AR (eds). *Caring for Muslim patients*. Radcliffe Medical Press, Abingdon, 2000.

CHAPTER 20

Mental Health on the Margins: Homelessness and Mental Disorder

Philip Timms and Adrian McLachlan

OVERVIEW

- Homelessness is the extreme end of the poverty spectrum and disproportionate numbers of mentally ill people are homeless; about 44% of homeless people have significant mental health problems

- Schizophrenia is the most common serious mental disorder; depression, alcohol dependence and personality disorders are also prevalent, and all are complicated by comorbid physical illness in many patients

- Homeless people have greatly increased difficulty accessing both physical and mental health services

- Treatment should be offered whenever possible, avoiding complex drug regimens, or drugs that might be abused or sold (e.g. benzodiazepines)

Box 20.1 Widely differing groups of people may become homeless

- Unemployed
- Middle-aged drinking men
- Teenage drug-abusers
- Patients with schizophrenia
- Children of homeless families
- Refugees and asylum seekers

Box 20.2 Spectrum of housing needs

- People living in existing households in unacceptable conditions
- Households sharing accommodation involuntarily (overcrowding)
- Imminent release from institutional accommodation (prison, hospital, local authority)
- Insecure tenure (holiday letting, tied accommodation, mortgage default)
- Accommodation for homeless people (hostels, night shelters, bed-and-breakfast)
- No shelter ('roofless', 'sleeping out' on streets, in parks or car parks)

People with mental disorders have always been marginalised and economically disadvantaged, and deprived inner-city areas have excessive rates of severe mental illness. Homelessness is the most extreme fringe of the poverty spectrum and disproportionate numbers of mentally ill people have been found consistently in homeless populations (Box 20.1).

What kind of homelessness?

Homeless people do not constitute a homogenous population: disparate groups are affected with widely differing needs. Mental health needs of people living in 'traditional' homeless lifestyles have elicited particular concern. We shall focus on the situation in the UK but very similar problems exist in the majority of Western industrialised countries (Box 20.2).

How many homeless people are there?

It is always difficult to say how many homeless people there are at any given time because there are several different ways of counting:

- National census every 10 years. The 1991 UK census counted around 3000 people sleeping out and 50,000 people living in homelessness hostels of some sort

- Number of households applying to local authority housing departments under the homelessness provision of the 1984 and 1996 Housing Acts ('homeless acceptances'). According to UK government data, the number of homeless households rose from about 100,000 in 1997 to a peak of 135,430 in 2003–4 (100,000 in temporary accommodation), with numbers falling gradually since. Unfortunately, this gives no details as to the precise housing status of those applicants and tends to exclude single homeless people as the criteria for vulnerability are much more easily met by parents with children

- Yearly counts of those sleeping out on the streets, usually carried out in September. These appear to show a substantial fall from the 1991 baseline of 3000 people sleeping out across England and Wales to 459 in 2005. However, street counts are necessarily an underestimate because they tend to miss those who sleep in isolated places or abandoned buildings. Charities working with homeless people claim a 10% increase in 'rough sleepers' from 2002 to 2005.

ABC of Mental Health, 2nd edition. Edited by T. Davies and T. Craig.
© 2009 Blackwell Publishing, ISBN: 978-0-7279-1639-6.

These methods of counting do help, but they omit those who live in hostels for homeless people and those who are 'hidden homeless', sleeping on friends' or relatives' floors. During 2002, a survey for the Greater London Authority found that the numbers of 'hidden homeless' people living in precarious accommodation where they have no legal right to stay was around 20 times greater than the hostel population of London. In the London boroughs of Southwark, Lambeth and Lewisham, the 2004 street count identified only 18 people who were sleeping out. This sounds like an admirably small number of people; however, during this period there were at least 500 places in generic hostels for homeless people, plus 36 places in projects specifically for homeless people with severe and enduring mental illness. And most of these beds were occupied most of the time.

Most homeless people do not stay permanently at any one point in the homelessness spectrum; they may move from street, to hostel, to a friend's place and then maybe back to the street again. An analysis of street homeless people in London in 2003 showed that, although the one-night street count number was 267, over the whole year 1547 different individuals had been recorded as homeless. So, homeless figures are probably best thought of in terms of a pyramid, with street homeless people forming the apex, followed sequentially down the pyramid by increasing numbers of hostel dwellers, and then by people in a variety of forms of insecure accommodation.

Black and minority ethnic (BME) groups

According to Shelter, a national charity for homeless people, BME households account for 32% of the 526,000 overcrowded households in England.

Refugees and asylum seekers

A survey in London in 2004 revealed that one-fifth of the beds in hostels for homeless people were occupied by refugees and asylum seekers (Box 20.3), mainly from African countries – most commonly Somalia, Eritrea and Ethiopia.

Box 20.3 **Pathways to homelessness**

Unemployment
  Lack of low-rent housing
    Marital break-up
      Death of a parent or carer
        Clashes with family/friends
          Leaving local authority care
            Leaving the armed forces
              Release from prison
                Episode of mental illness
                  'Failed' asylum application
Very few people choose to have no home

How many homeless people have mental health problems?

Compared with a point prevalence rate of 14% in the general population, 44% of homeless people have some kind of significant mental health problem such as schizophrenia, depression or personality disorder.

- Schizophrenia is massively over-represented in hostel populations, with point prevalence rates of 15–35% compared to a rate of <1% in the general population. In most surveys, it has been as common as alcohol dependence and is often unrecognised
- Depression has appeared to be less common than schizophrenia, although still with a high point prevalence of 5–16%. This is, of course, a mirror image of a normal general practice population where depression is common and schizophrenia unusual
- Alcohol misuse. Around 30% of homeless people are problem-drinkers: 49% of homeless men and 15% of homeless women are high-risk drinkers. Up to half the cases presenting to specialist teams in London have both a mental health problem and a drug or alcohol problem, so-called dual diagnosis
- Personality disorder. The point prevalence of personality disorder has been reported as being up to 50% of some homeless populations and is often a complicating factor in those presenting with substance abuse
- Post-traumatic stress disorder (PTSD). A survey found that asylum seekers who were in the process of having their claims considered were much more likely to present with PTSD than those whose claims had already been considered. The authors commented, 'The stresses of life in reception centres and the risk of being expelled from the country may contribute more to these admittances than experiences in the asylum seekers' countries of origin'. It is likely that a similar situation exists for such homeless people in the UK.

Pathways to care

Homeless people suffer from the same disorders as the general population, but there are major differences in both the pattern of disorder and in access to services. Although the absolute numbers are small, where they present in significant numbers they are perceived to place disproportionately large demands on local services, especially accident and emergency departments and psychiatric wards. The social support and physical resources that are necessary for health, and taken for granted by most people, simply do not exist. Contact with helping services, including primary care services, is likely to have been lost, and homeless people are unlikely to be receiving treatment.

Homelessness is often a consequence of severe mental illness

Major mental illness

Excessive rates of psychosis amongst the homeless have been reported since the 1950s and shelter for these vulnerable people was traditionally provided by hostels for the homeless. Although these institutions were supposed to afford only temporary accommodation, many people with chronic psychotic illnesses lived in them for many years. This may be because they were tolerant environments where, traditionally, very little 'rehabilitation pressure' was placed on residents. They served as *de facto* institutions, affording sanctuary but providing little adequate treatment, and producing the same institutional deficits as did the old asylums. Although the old, large, homeless hostels have gone, their smaller, higher quality modern counterparts still find themselves dealing with substantial numbers of people with major mental illness.

> Often ignored in research studies, both anxiety and depression are common in homeless people

Anxiety and depression

These disorders may result from the stresses of living without a home: they can be disabling, so trapping the individual in homelessness. Low-key support is often all that is needed and can produce dramatic improvements. Referral for psychotherapy or counselling should be made as appropriate on clinical grounds.

Substance misuse

Alcohol has been the traditional substance of misuse for homeless men, less so for women, and has often been the immediate precipitant of homelessness. Hence, the stigmatising stereotype that identifies all homeless people as alcoholics, despite the fact that psychosis is, in most UK studies, more common than alcoholism. Alcohol accounts for much of the small but striking number of homeless people with severe cognitive problems.

Drug misuse is an increasing problem amongst the growing proportion of young homeless people. Opiate addiction was historically unusual in this population but, over the last 10 years, has become a leading drug of choice as prices have dropped. Amphetamines and benzodiazepines are less commonly used than previously. The most common picture is of opportunistic polydrug abuse, often involving alcohol as well.

Dual diagnosis

Alcohol or drug abuse and psychosis are increasingly commonly found in the same individual. Such patients are particularly difficult to help, not only because of the multiplying effect of the disruption caused by each pathology, but also because they tend to fall between mainstream alcohol and psychiatric services.

Personality disorder

Although it seems to be generally accepted that many homeless people have a personality disorder, there are no good prevalence figures for the UK, possibly because of the difficulty of making this diagnosis on the basis of a one-off interview. However, those doing frontline work with homeless people have no doubt of the high prevalence amongst homeless people. Traditional long-term therapies may be difficult to organise in this group. However, cognitive behavioural therapy may be offered in hostel settings, and community teams can use multi-agency case conferences to coordinate the numerous services from various sectors that are often involved.

> Box 20.4 **Physical illness in homeless people**
>
> Offer to treat
> - Chest and other infections
> - Skin problems
> - Other conditions amenable to a short course of treatment
>
> Offer advice on
> - Contraception
> - Diet
> - Smoking and alcohol consumption
>
> Offer referral for
> - Chronic or serious physical conditions
> - Dental problems
> - Alcohol and drug misuse

Physical illness

Compared with the general population, homeless people suffer from considerably more untreated physical disease (Box 20.4). Chronic chest and skin disorders, traumatic injuries and dental problems predominate and may exacerbate anxiety and depression.

Barriers to care: professional attitudes

Stereotyping

Professionals are not immune to the popular stereotypes that portray the homeless as being alcoholic, personality disordered, feckless and as having chosen to live in this way. They often expect homeless patients to be both awkward and highly mobile.

'What difference can I make?'

The patient who is both homeless and mentally ill presents a multiplicity of needs. Usual interventions assume the presence of the social factors (housing, adequate nutrition and a social network) that make possible both health and treatment. Doctors may believe that they have nothing to offer when the absence of these factors seems to defeat any medical or psychiatric intervention.

> Difficulties treating homeless patients can produce a therapeutic nihilism that may not only prevent professionals from doing what they can, but also may even serve as a justification for neglect

Barriers to care: organisation of services

Multiple needs presenting at a single point in time

A homeless patient will often present with an array of problems, many of them outside the medical domain.

Inter-agency working

The multiple needs of the homeless mentally ill require the involvement of multiple agencies – health, social care and housing – in addition to specifically psychiatric input. This requires substantial inter-agency communication. Unfortunately, many health staff are unaware of the extensive network of local voluntary agencies providing support and care for homeless people.

Psychiatric 'no fixed address' (NFA) rotas

Many psychiatric units have a 'NFA rota' which allocates homeless patients to a duty psychiatric team. Unless this confers continuing responsibility for the patient, his or her care will be unnecessarily fragmented when, upon subsequent presentations, he or she is allocated to a different team.

Philosophies of care

Different agencies have differing philosophies of care. Most mental health services would consider that patients are unable to make informed choices when in the throes of a relapse of a severe mental illness. Some housing organisations take the view that people are always fully responsible for their choices and actions. This may lead to eviction if a disturbed or distressed patient is deemed, on account of his or her difficult behaviour, to have made a choice. To be fair, the inaccessibility of psychiatric help has often made it difficult for housing agencies to respond in any other way.

Local exclusionary practices

These include not allowing a person to register with a general practice if they do not have an address.

Temporary GP registration

Old notes are not requested from the health authority, reducing the standard and continuity of care.

Barriers to care: homeless lifestyles

Priorities

Both physical and psychiatric care rank low in homeless people's list of priorities. The demands of immediate survival needs – food, shelter, money – are usually more pressing than the need to see a doctor or a nurse.

Poor access to services

The GP is both gatekeeper and guide to most sources of psychiatric or psychological help. The homeless patient with no regular GP will often have to find his or her own way to these services, perhaps via the accident and emergency department. For obvious reasons, these departments are orientated towards brief intervention rather than continued involvement and advocacy.

Mobility

Mobility is as often forced upon the homeless as it is chosen. Although much of this movement is relatively local, primary and secondary care services may deny responsibility if catchment area boundaries are crossed.

Lack of social substrate for health or recovery

Effective medical interventions need an array of social factors (housing, adequate nutrition and a social network) to be in place.

Alienation

Homeless people have often been disappointed by statutory services. Their predicament makes demands that these agencies cannot easily meet, often provoking inadequate or even punitive responses. Hospitals and GPs are reluctant to take them on, benefits regulations seem specially designed to penalise them, council housing departments are only interested in homeless families and the very vulnerable. The police may move them on or arrest them for drunkenness or vagrancy. It is not surprising that homeless people are often suspicious and distrustful of services that see themselves as caring and helping.

Service provision: how to do it

Improve access

Conventional clinic times will not do for the homeless patient. It is more realistic to arrange meetings at times that fit in with their often irregular timetable. Even better is a drop-in service at a hostel or day centre where people can be seen quickly without appointment.

Provide information

Voluntary agencies provide most of the social care and support for homeless people. These commonly include hostels, day centres, sources of cheap or free food and clothing, alcohol counselling services and advice centres. Each primary care or mental health trust should obtain or create a directory of these services that is concise enough to be of use in a busy ward, general practice or accident and emergency department.

Access housing

Referral to the local authority social services or housing department (homeless persons unit) may lead to a considerable improvement in a patient's accommodation, but will often require the involvement of an advocate of some sort.

Find a key-worker or advocate

Treatment plans for homeless patients often fail because it is assumed that there is no carer with whom contact can be maintained. In fact, there is nearly always a person or organisation with whom they maintain contact and who should be informed. This might be a hostel or day-centre worker, an alcohol counsellor, a minister of religion, a social worker or a probation officer – the list is surprisingly long. Issues of confidentiality may arise, but can be overcome by obtaining the patient's written permission. Maintaining continuity of care (Box 20.5) is facilitated by producing an edited version of documents such as discharge summaries.

Prescribe cautiously

Whatever the temptation to prescribe benzodiazepines for someone who is obviously distressed – do not do it. Although most homeless patients use their medication responsibly, the benzodiazepines, chlormethiazole and procyclidine have a significant street value.

Do not prescribe abusable drugs

> ### Box 20.5 Maintaining continuity of care for homeless patients
>
> - Obtain, or create, a directory of local services for homeless people
> - Get to know the hostels that a patient uses – there may be several in a relatively small locality
> - Get to know the hostel workers and other people with whom patients may keep in contact
> - Be prepared to offer short-term courses of treatment
> - Use simple treatment regimens (single drugs, once daily doses)
> - Allow for patients' mobility – prepare a brief case summary for patients to carry with them or to be sent on request to other agencies
> - Be prepared to accept patients back into your care and to restart treatment
> - Build up trust – be accessible, flexible and sensitive to patients' priorities

> ### Box 20.6 Desirable service characteristics
>
> - 'Out there': provided in the community environment
> - Capable of rapid response
> - Informal: drop-in without appointment
> - Accessible: no complex, multistep or protracted referral procedures
> - Flexible: able to work in different environments in different styles
> - Multiskilled: able to deal with a range of medical and social needs
> - Collaborative: actively involved with other elements of the wider service network, particularly the voluntary sector
> - Responsive: able to change the service as circumstances and patients change

Lack of supervision makes it unwise to attempt alcohol or drug detoxification outside a well-organised hostel sick-bay, hospital or alcohol unit. Paradoxically, hostels for the homeless can be good places to prescribe antipsychotic medication. As there is often little pressure to achieve quick results, it is possible to start with low doses and increase slowly, minimising side effects and resistance to treatment. Adherence to any treatment regimen may be difficult because of lack of privacy, lack of secure storage, and erratic schedules for finding food or available shelter.

Use compulsory measures when necessary

Compulsory admission under the Mental Health Act is occasionally necessary, usually to treat an acute psychotic episode in which a patient becomes suicidal, violent or dangerous in other ways (such as setting fires). Prompt intervention and treatment could mean that a hostel is prepared to accept a patient back when he or she is discharged from hospital.

Conclusion

To provide a decent mental health service (Box 20.6) to homeless people may seem a daunting prospect. However, it is both possible and rewarding if it is coordinated as a part of more general housing

> ### Box 20.7 Practical steps in caring for homeless patients
>
> - If you want to know how many homeless people there are in your area, ask the local voluntary sector services. They will often be the sole providers of services in the area, although some local authority housing departments run accommodation projects for homeless people
> - Make sure you have a directory of local voluntary sector services for homeless people. If you do not know about them, you cannot use them
> - Ask your patient if he or she wants you to contact his or her hostel worker, key-worker, social worker or probation officer
> - Always consider psychosis as an explanation for disordered thinking, even when alcohol and drugs are involved
> - Consider the patient's hierarchy of needs. What is most important to him or her right now?
> - Always assume that a homeless patient will remain in your area; you are likely to try harder
> - Share the load if you can – do not struggle alone

and social provision (Box 20.7). Do not do what you cannot do, but make sure that you know someone who can. Homeless people are rewarding to treat and grateful to those who treat them professionally and with respect.

> ### Further information
>
> Crisis, 66 Commercial Street, London, E1 6LT
>   Telephone 0870 011 3335; fax: 0870 011 3336; email: enquiries@crisis.org.uk; http://www.crisis.org.uk
> Homeless Link, First Floor 10–13 Rushworth Street, London, SE1 0RB
>   Telephone 020 7960 3010; fax 020 7960 3011; http://www.homeless.org.uk
> Shelter, 88 Old Street, London, EC1V 9HU
>   Telephone 0845 458 4590; fax 020 7505 2030; email info@shelter.org.uk; http://shelter.org.uk

Further reading

Gill B, Meltzer H, Hinds K, Pettigrew M. *Psychiatric morbidity among homeless people. OPCS surveys of psychiatric morbidity in Great Britain. Report 7.* HMSO, London, 1996.

Haig R, Hibbert G. Where and when to detoxify single homeless drinkers. *BMJ* 1990; **301**: 848–9.

Iversen VC, Morken G. Differences in acute psychiatric admissions between asylum seekers and refugees. *Nordic J Psych* 2004; **58**: 465–70.

London Housing Foundation. *Survey of homelessness sector services provided to asylum seeker and refugee clients.* Broadway London, London, 2004. http://www.broadwaylondon.org/broadwayvoice/policy/refugees_final_report.pdf

Office of National Statistics. *Substance misuse and mental disorder among homeless people in Glasgow.* ONS, London, 2000.

Palmer G. *The numbers of hidden homeless and other people in housing need – A report for the GLA.* New Policy Institute, London, 2004. www.npi.org.uk/reports/homelessness%20gla.pdf

CHAPTER 21

Mental Health and the Law

Humphrey Needham-Bennett

OVERVIEW

- The Mental Health Act 2007 amends the previous, 1983, Act and introduces a single legal category of mental disorder, defined as any disorder or disability of the mind

- Most sections of the Act remain unchanged in relation to compulsory detention of patients; section 25A (supervised discharge) has been replaced by supervised community treatment; the roles of some of the personnel specified in the Act have changed

- Maintaining confidentiality is a common law duty, and is required by the Human Rights Act 1998; patient-identifiable information may be disclosed to third parties in strictly defined circumstances

- Under the Mental Capacity Act 2005, patients aged 16 and over are presumed to have capacity to make their own decisions unless shown otherwise; capacity depends on the patient's ability to understand, retain and use information relevant to a decision, and communicate that decision

All doctors and many other healthcare professionals have legitimate powers, responsibilities and duties in relation to the care and treatment of their patients. Some of these, such as the common law duty of care and doctrine of necessity, apply to all patients, whereas others arise from statute law and apply specifically to those with mental disorders. This chapter provides a summary of the law applying to the treatment of people with mental disorders in England and Wales. It deals with how consent to treatment may be determined and considers the common law duty of confidence.

Mental Health Acts

Whilst most treatment of mental disorder is undertaken voluntarily, or in an emergency under the common law, the Mental Health Acts 1983 and 2007 can allow compulsory admission and treatment under some circumstances ('sectioning'). Article 5 of the Human Rights Act 1998 details a right to liberty but includes provision for the detention of persons of unsound mind.

ABC of Mental Health, 2nd edition. Edited by T. Davies and T. Craig. © 2009 Blackwell Publishing, ISBN: 978-0-7279-1639-6.

The Mental Health Act 2007, implemented fully from 2008 onwards, amends the provisions of the 1983 Act. However, as many sections remain unchanged, a description of the 1983 Act will be used as an introduction to the current position (Box 21.1).

The 1983 Act allowed for compulsory admission to a registered hospital facility for assessment where the patient was believed to be suffering, or for treatment if known to be suffering, from one of a set of mental disorders (Box 21.2). For a patient to be admitted for treatment, the type of disorder was defined and was of a nature or degree which made it appropriate for him to receive medical treatment in hospital that was necessary for the health or safety of the patient or for the protection of others. Though mental illness was undefined, the definitions of mental impairment and psychopathic disorder included a disorder of behaviour, and both must have been considered treatable to warrant admission to hospital (the 'treatability' condition).

Compulsory admission

Section 2 allows for compulsory admission for assessment and treatment for up to 28 days, and section 3 for treatment for up to six months. Both require recommendations by two doctors (one being approved under section 12 of the Act, and the other should have prior knowledge of the patient). An application for admission is normally made by an approved mental health professional (AMHP), part of his or her role being to ensure that hospital treatment is necessary. Detention for treatment (section 3) may be extended under section 20 subject to a recommendation from the responsible clinician (RC, clinician in charge of the patient's treatment).

Article 5(4) of the Human Rights Act requires speedy decisions relating to lawfulness of detention of persons of unsound mind. The RC, the nearest relative, the hospital managers (the legal detaining authority), and the Mental Health Review Tribunal can remove the liability to be detained. The burden of proof is with the detaining authority.

Emergency admission

Section 4 permits admission in cases of urgent necessity. One doctor and a social worker or the nearest relative may compel admission. Assessment by a second approved doctor may 'convert' this to a section 2.

- **Definition of mental disorder.** Single definition without subcategories applies to all sections of the Act. Excludes drug or alcohol dependence, and learning disability unless accompanied by abnormally aggressive or seriously irresponsible behaviour
- **Criteria for detention.** Patient suffering a mental disorder of a nature or degree to warrant detention (section 2), or to receive medical treatment (section 3) in hospital. Detention must be in the interests of the patient's health or safety or for the protection of others, and appropriate medical treatment must be available
- **Appropriate medical treatment.** Detention for treatment will be permitted only if the patient is able to receive 'appropriate medical treatment'. This replaces the so-called treatability test of the 1983 Act
- **Approved mental health professional (AMHP).** This role permits a broad range of mental health professionals (but excluding doctors) to undertake the statutory duties formerly undertaken by the approved social worker (ASW)
- **Responsible clinician (RC).** The approved clinician in overall charge of a patient's care and treatment. This role replaces that of the responsible medical officer (RMO) and again permits a broader group of senior mental health professionals to undertake the statutory duties under the Act
- **Approved clinician.** A clinician of any mental health profession who is approved as having special expertise in managing mental disorders. Approved clinicians may take charge of aspects of the patient's care. All responsible clinicians must be approved
- **Community treatment orders (CTO).** Permits patients at high risk of relapsing due to non-compliance with treatment to live in the community while subject to the treatment requirements of sections 3 and 37 of the Act. Replaces section 25A of previous legislation
- **Section 136.** Patients may be transferred from one place of safety to another
- **Nearest relative.** Civil partners to be recognised as nearest relatives. A patient may apply to a court to displace his or her nearest relative
- **Independent mental health advocates.** To be available to all detained patients in hospital and community

Mental Health Act 1983
- Mental illness: undefined
- Psychopathic disorder: a persistent disorder or disability of mind (whether or not including significant impairment of intelligence), which results in abnormally aggressive or seriously irresponsible conduct
- Mental impairment: arrested or incomplete development of mind, which includes significant impairment of intelligence and social functioning and is associated with abnormally aggressive or seriously irresponsible conduct
- Severe mental impairment: arrested or incomplete development of mind, which includes severe impairment of intelligence and social functioning and is associated with abnormally aggressive or seriously irresponsible conduct

Mental Health Act 2007
- Mental disorder: any disorder or disability of the mind. This single definition with no subcategories applies throughout the Act

Treating patients

Treatment may be subject to informed consent, under the common law, or under a section of the Mental Health Act. All treatments must be in the patient's best interest.

Common law: in an emergency, treatment can be given under the common law principles of duty of care and doctrine of necessity

Section 57 applies to certain irreversible treatments (e.g. psychosurgery) that require both consent and a second opinion. Section 58 covers treatment requiring consent or a second opinion (e.g. administration of medicine after three months of treatment). Second opinion approved doctors (SOADs) are appointed by the Mental Health Act Commission to examine the patient and grant or withhold the consent for treatment. As sections 57 and 58 do not cover treatment needed immediately (emergency treatment necessary to save life, prevent serious deterioration, alleviate suffering, or necessary to prevent violent or dangerous behaviour), these are permitted under section 62. Section 62 allows treatment of recalled patients.

Section 63 concerns treatment which does not require the patient's consent (administration of medication within the first three months of detention). This section also covers general nursing care, and other psychological, occupational and social therapies. Technically, these treatments must be authorised by the RC, though in practice it is self-evident that they could not be undertaken without the patient's consent or cooperation.

Part 4 of the Act only allows for treatment of physical disorders that give rise to mental disorder when it is necessary to treat the mental disorder (i.e. thyrotoxicosis, neurosyphilis).

If the patient is already receiving care as a hospital inpatient (this does not include patients in accident and emergency departments), he or she may be prevented from leaving hospital by a doctor nominated by the RC, under section 5(2), or by a suitably qualified nurse, under section 5(4). Formal assessment for detention under sections 2 or 3 should then follow.

Section 136 allows the police to bring a person from a public place to a designated 'place of safety' if it appears he or she is suffering from a mental disorder and is in immediate need of care or control.

Section 135 allows a magistrate (on advice from a social worker) to authorise police to convey a person from a private dwelling to a place of safety when believed to be suffering from a mental disorder.

Consent to treatment

Adults (here taken as 16 and over) are assumed to have capacity unless demonstrated otherwise. The key questions are whether the patient can:

- Understand the information relevant to the decision
- Retain it
- Use or weigh the information as part of the process of making the decision
- Communicate his or her decision, by whatever means.

Unexpected, unwise and even perverse decisions do not necessarily mean that the patient lacks capacity.

Consent should be seen as a process and not as a single event. Patients are able to change their mind and can withdraw consent at any stage

---

For incapacitated adults, no-one else can give consent on their behalf. Doctors are required to act in the patient's 'best interest', and this goes further than just medical interest and includes factors such as his or her wishes and beliefs when competent, and his or her spiritual and religious welfare. Good practice will involve wide consultation in determining best interest (Box 21.3).

If a patient aged 18 and over lacks capacity but has indicated clearly (in the past whilst competent) that he or she would refuse treatment in certain situations (an advance directive or advance decision), the doctor must abide by that refusal. The Mental Capacity Act 2005 came into force in England and Wales in 2007, and helps clarify these common law procedures. All patients are presumed to have capacity to make decisions about their lives unless shown otherwise; they may lack capacity for some decisions while retaining it for others. The Act sets out the procedures for determining capacity (e.g. in specified circumstances, when a decision needs to be made) and introduces a lasting power of attorney: patients may choose someone to make decisions on their behalf, not only about financial matters but also personal welfare. It is the duty

---

Box 21.3 **Valid consent**

- Being detained under the Mental Health Act does not imply inability to consent
- Consent may be implied (offering arm for venepuncture), verbal or non-verbal or written
- A signature on a consent form does not prove consent
- An explanation of the proposed treatment must be understandable and appropriate to the circumstances
- Good practice requires the discussion about the proposed treatment, alternatives, risks and benefits, to be recorded fully
- Retaining information only for a short period does not prevent a decision
- Consent has to be voluntary and not under duress or undue influence from health professionals, family or friends
- Patients can give partial consent (e.g. refusal of a blood transfusion during operation)

---

of all healthcare professionals, not merely psychiatrists, to assess competence.

Children

The Mental Health Act applies to patients of all ages, including children. Below the age of 16 the doctor must ascertain that the child understands fully what is involved. A parent or legal guardian should be involved in this discussion. Where the child is under 16 and does not have capacity, someone with parental responsibility must give consent on the child's behalf unless they cannot be reached in an emergency. If a competent child consents to treatment, a parent cannot override that consent. However, if a competent child under 16 refuses, a parent can consent though treatment in such circumstances may be difficult or impossible. The 2007 Act removes this provision for 16–18 year olds.

Supervised discharge

Section 25A was inserted into the Mental Health Act by the Mental Health (Patients in the community) Act 1995 to target so-called revolving door patients – those who are compulsorily admitted, treated, improve, discharged, fail to comply with the treatment plan and relapse, leading to readmission. This section was rescinded by the 2007 Act and replaced by community treatment orders, section 17 (Box 21.1).

A patient recalled to hospital may be treated under section 62A of the Act.

Treatment of mentally disordered offenders (MDOs)

Both Magistrate and Crown Courts can make a 'hospital order' under section 37 on the advice of two doctors. The person then becomes a hospital inpatient instead of receiving any other legal sanction. The seriousness of the offence and the degree of illness and risk will determine what level of security is afforded the patient when he or she is transferred to a hospital facility. The provisions afforded by section 37 are broadly similar to those of section 3, and the patient may be discharged from hospital by the RC on satisfactory response to treatment.

Crown Courts have an additional power to impose a restrictionorder under section 41. In considering whether to impose a restriction order, the court will consider the nature of the offence, previous offending behaviour and the risk of committing further offences, and the need to protect the public from serious harm. Section 41 makes discharge from hospital possible only through the Home Office or the Mental Health Review Tribunal. These bodiesmay discharge patients conditionally, and conditions may relate to place of residence or treatment. While medication cannot be given compulsorily in the community, a failure to comply with the conditions of the discharge may result in a recall to hospital.

Sections 35, 36 and 38 allow courts in certain situations to hospitalise a defendant to allow an inpatient assessment (and treatment for sections 36 and 38) of mental disorder. The court will receive medical reports on diagnosis or response to treatment, and use this information in sentencing or making a hospital order.

Mentally disordered prisoners

Section 47 and 48 allow transfer of sentenced and unsentenced prisoners to hospital for treatment. The Home Office normally imposes a restriction order under section 49 (similar to section 41), so that when the prisoner no longer requires treatment in hospital, he or she is returned to prison.

Probation orders

Outpatient psychiatric treatment may be provided under a probation order imposed by the court. An order can be made only if the patient agrees to the conditions imposed. In the event of a patient breaching the conditions of the order, he or she may be returned to court for an alternative sanction.

Confidentiality

Patients have a right to expect information about them to be held in confidence by their doctors, and this is central to the trust between doctor and patient. Confidentiality is underpinned by the common law duty of confidence, and is expressed in the Data Protection Act 1998 and the Human Rights Act 1998 (Article 8, right to privacy and family life). It is reinforced by professional guidance (e.g. from the General Medical Council (GMC)), the government's Health Department and the doctor's contract of employment. Each NHS Trust is required to appoint a Caldicott Guardian to ensure that the sharing of patient-identifiable information is justified, necessary and lawful.

Police do not have a general right of access to health records. Disclosure must be with the patient's consent, be justified by an overriding public interest (e.g. prevention of serious crime) or be required by statutory obligations or court order (Box 21.4). Information disclosed should be the minimum necessary, and the

---

Box 21.4 Patient-identifiable information may be passed on to others in the following circumstances

- With patient's consent
- Under statutory law (e.g. Children Acts 1989 and 2004, Road Traffic Act 1988). Section 115 of the Crime & Disorder Act 1998 permits but does not require disclosure
- Under court order, including a coroner's court
- When the patient is incapacitated and the doctor is acting in his or her best interest
- When disclosure may be justified in the public interest (where the benefit to an individual or to society of disclosure outweighs the public and the patient's interest in keeping the information confidential). The doctor may breach confidentiality when the failure to disclose information would expose the patient or someone else to a risk of death or serious harm
- Formal police enquiry under the Data Protection Act
- On request from bodies with statutory investigative powers (GMC, Audit Commission, Health Service Ombudsman)

---

patient should be informed of the disclosure unless to do so would place a criminal investigation, or third parties, in jeopardy.

Patients have a legal right of access to their medical records in whatever medium these are held, unless the information is likely to cause serious harm to their mental health or cause serious harm to another person. If the medical record contains third-party information (i.e. not from a healthcare professional), there is a duty to seek that person's consent for disclosure, or remove his or her contribution from the information provided.

Multi-agency public protection arrangements (MAPPA)

This represents a coming together of police, probation and prison services to manage violent and sexual offenders. The MAPPA deal with three groups of offenders at different levels of risk:
- All registered sex offenders
- All violent and non-registered sex offenders sentenced to more than 12 months of imprisonment, those made subject to section 37 of the Mental Health Act, and those found not guilty by reason of insanity
- Others believed to pose a risk of serious harm.

The Criminal Justice Act 2003 imposes on each healthcare trust, a 'duty to cooperate' with the MAPPA. This duty does not diminish the duty of confidentiality to the patient.

Voting rights

The Representation of the People Act 2000 provides that a person is entitled to vote if they are included on the Register of Electors. A person will be barred from voting if he or she does not have the requisite capacity, or if he or she is an offender detained in a mental hospital. Generally, residents in mental hospitals may register to vote while inpatients.

National Assistance Act 1948

Section 47 of this Act allows for a patient to be removed from his or her dwelling place to a suitable premises, most often a hospital, if all the following conditions are met:
- Living in unsanitary conditions
- Suffering from serious chronic disease, or aged or infirm, or physically incapacitated
- Not receiving proper care and attention.

The doctor, usually a public health physician, makes a report to this effect, which then requires approval from the local court.

Testamentary capacity

A doctor may assist the court in determining testamentary capacity, that is the capacity to make a legally valid will. Case law (Banks versus Goodfellow 1870, LR 5 QB 549) establishes four key tests for determining this capacity. The person making the will must understand:
- The nature of the act of making it
- The effect of doing so

- The extent of the property disposed of, and
- The claims other persons may have upon the estate.

Further reading

Davies T. Consent to treatment. *Psych Bull* 1997; **21**: 200–1.

Department for Constitutional Affairs. *Mental Capacity Act 2005. Code of practice*. The Stationcry Office, London, 2007. http://www.dca.gov.uk/legal-policy/mental-capacity/mca-cp.pdf

Department for Education and Skills. *The multi-agency public protection arrangements (the MAPPA)*. DfES, London, 2003. http://www.dfes.gov.uk/childrenandfamilies/docs/MAPPA%20&%20DTC%20summary%20Nov%2003%20-%202.doc

Department of Health. *Confidentiality: NHS code of practice*. DH, London, 2003. http://www.dh.gov.uk/en/Publicationsandstatistics/Publications/PublicationsPolicyAndGuidance/DH_4069253

Office of Public Sector Information. *Mental Capacity Act 2005*. OPSI, London, 2007. http://www.opsi.gov.uk/acts/acts2005/20050009.htm

Office of Public Sector Information. *Mental Health Act 2007*. OPSI, London, 2007. http://www.opsi.gov.uk/acts/acts2007/ukpga_20070012_en_2#pt1

UK Council of Caldicott Guardians. *The Caldicott Guardian manual 2006*. Department of Health, London, 2006. http://www.dh.gov.uk/en/Publicationsandstatistics/Publications/PublicationsPolicyAndGuidance/DH_062722

CHAPTER 22

Drug Treatments in Mental Health

Soumitra R Pathare and Carol Paton

OVERVIEW

- All antidepressants are equally effective and show similar onset of action in treating moderate or severe depression; choice depends on side effects or potential for interactions
- All antipsychotic drugs are equally effective in treating positive symptoms of schizophrenia; atypical antipsychotics have some efficacy against negative symptoms; clozapine is more effective than other drugs for 'treatment-resistant' schizophrenia
- Mood stabilisers vary in their relative ability to control elevated or depressed mood in bipolar affective disorder
- Adherence to drug treatment reduces both frequency and severity of relapses of mental disorder
- Adherence to prescribed treatment is poor with almost all psychotropic drugs; steps to improve adherence involve increasing the patient's comprehension (understanding of treatment), comfort (by minimising side effects) and collaboration (involvement in treatment decisions)

Medication may be considered for treatment of many mental disorders, and is the mainstay of treatment in some. This chapter takes a broad view of the factors affecting the choice and effectiveness of common drugs used to treat mental disorders. Specific issues of diagnosis and treatment are dealt with in earlier chapters in this book.

Antidepressant medication

Antidepressant drugs are no more effective than placebo in treating mild depression. Problem-solving, self-help, bibliotherapy (use of self-help manuals) and exercise are all more effective in this group of patients. As the severity of depression increases, antidepressants are more likely to be helpful.

All antidepressants are equally effective, and no single drug has been shown to have a more rapid onset of action than another. The choice of antidepressant is dictated by a combination of factors including the clinical presentation, the patient's physical health, the anticipated side effect profile (Box 22.1) and the prescriber's preferences.

ABC of Mental Health, 2nd edition. Edited by T. Davies and T. Craig.
© 2009 Blackwell Publishing, ISBN: 978-0-7279-1639-6.

Box 22.1 **Disadvantages of different classes of antidepressant medication**

Tricyclic antidepressants (TCAs)
- Prominent anticholinergic side effects such as dry mouth, blurred vision, constipation, postural hypotension and urinary retention
- Need to start with a small dose and increase gradually
- Weight gain is a substantial problem
- More serious side effects include
  - Cardiac arrhythmias
  - Seizures
  - Depression of central nervous system (potentiated by alcohol)
  - Toxicity in overdose

Selective serotonin reuptake inhibitors (SSRIs)
- Development of serotonergic syndrome (characterised by headache, gastrointestinal upset, nausea and anxiety)
- Lack of sedation
- Potential for interactions with other drugs (warfarin, phenytoin, etc.)
- Some distressing side effects (especially sexual dysfunction)
- Increased risk of upper gastrointestinal bleeding when taken with NSAIDs (most problematic in the very old)

Venlafaxine
- Poorly tolerated in primary care patients (not recommended for first-line use)
- Troublesome side effects (sweating, headache)
- More toxic on overdose than SSRIs (safer than TCAs)
- More cardiotoxic than SSRIs

Mirtazapine
- Sedative
- Weight gain

Monoamine oxidase inhibitors (MAOIs)
- Main drawback is dangerous interaction with tyramine-rich foods and sympathomimetic drugs, which can lead to hypertensive crisis
- Anticholinergic side effects
- Hepatotoxicity
- Need for washout period

Types of depression

Certain types of depression respond better to particular classes of drug, e.g. atypical depressive illness and monoamine oxidase inhibitors (MAOIs).

Suicide risk

Overall, selective serotonin reuptake inhibitors (SSRIs) are safer than tricyclics in overdose, with dosulepin (dothiepin) having been found to be the most toxic. As suicide risk in any given patient is difficult to predict, SSRIs should be the first choice of treatment in all cases of depressive illness. The most effective way to prevent suicide is to:

• Identify those at greatest risk
• Give small supplies to patients at risk
• Use a therapeutic dose of any antidepressant, not a small dose of a 'safe' one.

Psychotic depression

The presence of delusions in depressive illness usually predicts a poor response to antidepressants alone. Addition of an antipsychotic drug will greatly improve the outcome. The dose required is usually lower than for the treatment of schizophrenia.

Dose and duration of antidepressant treatment

Many depressed patients are given too small a dose of antidepressant for too short a time, leading to poor response, repeated relapses and increased morbidity. About 70% of patients respond to the first antidepressant administered if it is given at a therapeutic dose for an adequate period (minimum 6–8 weeks).

If there is no response, and adherence is not in doubt, the dose should be increased if tolerated or the antidepressant changed to one from a different class. The short washout period of mirtazapine is useful in transferring to or from other antidepressants. A further 10–15% of patients will respond to an alternative drug. If the response is still inadequate, specialist referral is appropriate.

For a single episode of depression, treatment should be continued after remission of symptoms for at least six months in younger patients and at least two years in elderly patients (Box 22.2). If there are recurrent episodes then a maintenance dose of antidepressant should be considered for at least three years. The importance of adherence should be emphasised, along with the risk of relapse if treatment is stopped prematurely: 65% of patients who stop treatment relapse within a year, compared with 15% of those who continue drug treatment. People with chronic or treatment-resistant depression may benefit from cognitive behavioural therapy (CBT) in addition to antidepressant drugs.

People with depression often self-medicate with herbal remedies, the most important of which is St John's Wort. Although effective for mild or moderate depression, St John's Wort does not seem to be useful in severe depression. It is a potent enzyme inducer and interacts with many drugs (such as warfarin, protease inhibitors, cyclosporin, etc.) rendering them ineffective. It can cause serotonergic syndrome when used alongside SSRIs.

Antipsychotic medication

As with the antidepressants, no individual antipsychotic drug, except for clozapine, has been shown to be any more effective than another in treating schizophrenia (Box 22.3). All are effective at treating so-called positive symptoms (hallucinations, delusions and thought disorder). Traditional antipsychotics have limited efficacy

---

Box 22.2 Treatment of depression

First-line treatment
• Mild depression does not respond well to antidepressant drugs. Advise on self-help, exercise; offer problem-solving and a review appointment
• Moderate/severe depression: offer an antidepressant drug. Generic SSRIs are cheap, generally better tolerated than alternatives and easy to use
• Review after 1–2 weeks to exclude the emergence of increased agitation and suicidal thoughts

Second-line treatment
• If no response by 4–6 weeks, consider increasing the dose or switching to an alternative antidepressant (including venlafaxine)
• If no response to second drug, consider referral to secondary care

Augmentation
• Options include addition of lithium or a second antidepressant

Continuation and maintenance
• Treat for six months after remission for a single episode and at least three years if multiple episodes
• Ensure patients are aware of the risk of discontinuation symptoms and how to minimise them (decrease dose slowly at the end of treatment)

Box 22.3 Clozapine

• Recommended for treatment-resistant schizophrenia; 60% of patients respond
• Treatment must be initiated by a consultant psychiatrist; may be prescribed by a general practitioner via shared care arrangement
• Lacks extrapyramidal side effects
• Main side effects: sedation, hypersalivation, seizures
• 3% incidence of neutropenia, hence need for full blood count, weekly at first then at longer intervals if patient haematologically stable
• Avoid other drugs with myelosuppressive potential, such as depot antipsychotics, sulphonamides, chloramphenicol and cytotoxic drugs

---

against the negative symptoms (e.g. withdrawal, lack of volition), and the newer drugs (clozapine, olanzapine, risperidone, quetiapine, amisulpride and aripiprazole) have some advantages in this respect.

The older, traditional drugs are usually differentiated by the degree of sedation they produce, with chlorpromazine being the most sedative and trifluoperazine the least. The converse tends to be true for antipsychotic potency, with the more sedative drugs being less potent than their non-sedative alternatives. The high-potency compounds are used primarily for treating acutely psychotic adults, whereas the low-potency compounds are used when agitation is prominent or their sedative effects are desirable.

In elderly patients, high-potency compounds can produce severe extrapyramidal side effects (EPSEs) (see Box 22.8), whereas low-potency drugs can lead to troublesome postural hypotension. All of these drugs are associated with increased morbidity in elderly people because of their adverse effects on mobility. Risperidone and

Box 22.4 **Atypical antipsychotics: NICE guidance**

- Choice of antipsychotic should be made jointly by the prescriber and the patient
- Atypicals should be considered in the choice of first-line treatment (less extrapyramidal side effects, EPSEs)
- Patients unresponsive to two different antipsychotics (used sequentially) should receive clozapine
- Atypical and typical drugs should not be co-prescribed, except during changeover from one to the other
- Advance directives outlining patients' wishes about future drug treatment should be developed

Box 22.5 **Other side effects of antipsychotic medication**

Common side effects
- Extrapyramidal side effects (mainly typical antipsychotics)
- Sedation
- Anticholinergic effects made worse by antimuscarinic drugs (such as procyclidine)
- Prolactin-related side effects such as amenorrhoea and gynaecomastia (typicals, risperidone and amisulpride)
- Sexual dysfunction
- Weight gain, hyperlipidaemia and diabetes: regular screening is essential
- Photosensitivity (mainly chlorpromazine)
- Increased risk of stroke in elderly patients with dementia (most associated with risperidone and olanzapine but likely to occur with all antipsychotics)

Rare side effects
- Epileptic seizures
- Neuroleptic malignant syndrome (more common with typicals)
- Bone marrow suppression
- Abnormalities in cardiac conduction (QT interval prolongation)
- Rare association with unexplained sudden death

Box 22.6 **Neuroleptic malignant syndrome**

A rare, but life-threatening, condition that can occur with any antipsychotic drug, irrespective of dose. Prompt identification is vital as patient needs specialist intensive medical treatment. It is most common when starting treatment or increasing the dose

Presentation
- Fever
- Muscular rigidity
- Confusion and impaired consciousness
- Autonomic instability (excessive sweating, labile blood pressure, tachycardia)
- Grossly raised serum creatinine kinase

Management
- Stop antipsychotic drugs immediately
- Manage psychotic disturbance with benzodiazepines or other sedatives
- Monitor cardiovascular and renal function
- Admission to intensive medical treatment unit may be required
- After recovery from acute syndrome, consider cautiously reinstating antipsychotic drugs

Box 22.7 **Depot antipsychotic preparations**

- No additional efficacy over oral preparations
- Not recommended for use during the acute phase of an illness
- If patient has responded to an oral preparation of a particular drug, try a depot preparation of the same drug or another drug from the same class
- If reducing dose, gradual reduction (10% of dose at a time) is recommended
- Only useful in non-adherent patients who forget to take, or dislike taking, tablets on a daily basis
- Of limited use with other causes of non-adherence, as patients can default on depot preparations as well
- Risperidone is the only atypical available in depot form. It is formulated as an aqueous suspension and can only be given in three doses (25 mg, 37.5 mg or 50 mg at fortnightly intervals)

olanzapine (and possibly all antipsychotics) have been associated with stroke in elderly patients with dementia, and they should not be used to treat behavioural problems in this patient group.

Atypical antipsychotics are better tolerated with respect to EPSEs (Box 22.4). Individual drugs can cause sedation (olanzapine), postural hypotension (risperidone, quetiapine), prolactin-related side effects (risperidone, amisulpride) and anticholinergic side effects (olanzapine, quetiapine) (Box 22.5 and 22.6).

Response to antipsychotic treatment

Antipsychotics have a general calming effect and are useful in reducing arousal in the first few days of treatment. The antipsychotic effect is more variable in onset, though as a general rule it is unusual to see much improvement before a week, and most of the therapeutic gain tends to build up during the first six weeks. A therapeutic dose for an adequate period of time (such as risperidone 4 mg/day for six weeks) will produce a good response in one-third of patients, a partial response in a further third, and minimal or no response in the remainder.

The conventional duration of treatment for a first episode of schizophrenia is one to two years after complete remission of symptoms. For repeated episodes, it is recommended that treatment is continued for at least five years and in some instances for life.

Dose of antipsychotic drugs

There is no evidence that high doses lead to a more rapid response or to improved efficacy in most patients who receive them. They lead to a high incidence of side effects and may be associated with sudden cardiac death. The Royal College of Psychiatrists' consensus statement on the use of high-dose antipsychotics urges careful consideration and documentation of all the relevant facts before embarking on the cautious use of high-dose or regimens of multiple antipsychotics (Box 22.7).

Combination antipsychotics

Combinations of antipsychotic drugs should not be used generally as there is no evidence that this practice reduces side effects. The associated risks are poorly quantified but include increased mortality. Exceptions to this rule include patients who are changing from one antipsychotic to another, and those with treatment-resistant illness who are only partially responsive to clozapine (patients in the latter group should be dealt with by specialist units).

Anticholinergic medication

Anticholinergic (strictly, antimuscarinic) drugs are used to relieve the EPSEs of antipsychotic drugs (Box 22.8). Extrapyramidal side effects can be frightening and socially stigmatising, and many patients refuse further antipsychotic drugs as a result. Anticholinergics are often required with older antipsychotic drugs, and patients should be reviewed with a view to prescribing an atypical antipsychotic instead. Patients prescribed atypicals do not usually (but may) require anticholinergics.

Anticholinergic drugs produce a pleasurable 'buzz', which encourages misuse and dependence. Other side effects include drowsiness, dry mouth, blurred vision and constipation. In elderly patients they can sometimes lead to an acute confusional state. They also interfere with the treatment of glaucoma, and cause acute urinary retention in patients with prostatic hypertrophy. Hence, for most patients, anticholinergics should be prescribed only in the presence of obvious EPSEs.

Antianxiety medication

Mild anxiety is best treated by non-drug means such as CBT, or training in anxiety management or relaxation techniques. Benzodiazepines can be useful in treating acute distress or agitation and acute generalised anxiety (Box 22.9), but should not be used to treat panic disorder. Tolerance to their effects can develop within days to weeks and they have a high potential for producing dependence (Box 22.10). They should not be prescribed for longer than four weeks. Both generalised anxiety disorder and panic disorder respond best to CBT. If this is not available or the patient prefers, SSRIs are effective and reasonably well tolerated. It may be necessary to start at a low dose (half the dose used for depression) and titrate up slowly.

Zopiclone, zaleplon and zolpidem are non-benzodiazepine hypnotics ('Z-hypnotics'). They are no more effective than benzodiazepines and no less likely to lead to dependence. Disturbed sleep is a common presenting problem in depression, anxiety and alcohol

---

Box 22.8 **Extrapyramidal side effects (EPSEs) of antipsychotic medication**

Parkinsonian syndrome
- Presentation: mask-like face, tremor at rest, rigidity, shuffling gait, motor retardation
- Differentiate from withdrawal and apathy of schizophrenia syndrome
- Treatment: anticholinergic drugs

Dystonias
- Presentation: dystonic movements primarily affecting face, neck and tongue and, rarely, the trunk and limbs. Oculogyric crisis
- Treatment: anticholinergic drugs, by parenteral route if severe

Akathisia
- Presentation: psychomotor restlessness described by patients as a constant urge to move and an inability to sit still
- Differentiate from agitation of schizophrenia
- Treatment: poor response to anticholinergic drugs. Reduce dose of antipsychotic drug if possible. Small doses of benzodiazepine or propranolol or cyproheptadine may help (seek specialist advice)

Tardive dyskinesia
- A late side effect, usually apparent after many years of drug treatment but can occur sooner. Not associated with any particular drug and not dose-dependent. Increasing age and cumulative dose are risk factors
- Presentation: involuntary movements affecting the face and the limbs. Sucking, smacking of lips, choreoathetoid movements of tongue. Choreiform movements in limbs. Rarely affects truncal muscles
- Treatment: gradually reduce dose of antipsychotic drug. Consider replacing with an atypical antipsychotic

---

Box 22.9 **Prescribing benzodiazepines**

Do
- Identify the cause of anxiety or insomnia and treat appropriately
- Encourage patients to consider non-drug methods of treatment
- Reserve benzodiazepines for anxiety or insomnia that is severe and disabling
- Use the smallest effective dose for the shortest period of time
- Use a short-acting benzodiazepine or 'Z-hypnotic' for insomnia
- Use long-acting benzodiazepine for daytime relief of severe anxiety
- Warn patients about dangers of dependence

Do not
- Prescribe for more than 2–4 weeks
- Give 'routine' or repeat prescriptions
- Prescribe to patients who are liable to dependence

Box 22.10 **Side effects of benzodiazepines**

- Daytime drowsiness
- Impaired memory and concentration
- Impaired reaction times: patients should be warned of dangers of driving or operating machinery
- Potentates depressive effects of alcohol on central nervous system: can lead to accidental overdose
- Respiratory depression, especially in elderly patients and those with chronic airway disease
- Elderly patients prescribed benzodiazepines are more likely to have falls resulting in fractures
- Abrupt discontinuation can precipitate epileptic seizures
- Rarely, psychosis may occur during withdrawal

misuse, so it is important to identify and treat the cause. Insomnia after a life event such as bereavement, or associated with extraneous factors such as noise and shift work, is also common. Many patients with a severe physical illness and pain complain of poor sleep. In all such cases, a short course of hypnotics should be prescribed only if the sleep disturbance is very severe, disabling and causing extreme distress. Hypnotics started during a brief hospital admission should be stopped on discharge.

Mood-stabilising medication

Lithium

The decision to use mood stabilisers should be taken only after consideration of the individual risk factors for any given patient (Box 22.11). As a general rule, prophylaxis should be considered if two episodes of mood disorder (one being hypomania) occur within a two-year period.

When used in bipolar disorder, the risk of early relapse of mania after discontinuation of lithium is high (higher than that expected from the natural course of the disorder). For this reason, it is probably wise not to start treatment in bipolar illness unless it is intended to continue it for at least three years. Major psychiatric illness is associated with a 30-fold increase in the suicide rate. Maintenance treatment with lithium reduces mortality from suicide in bipolar disorder to the same level as that seen in the general population. There is no convincing evidence that mortality from other causes is increased.

Side effects tend to be directly related to plasma levels of lithium and are infrequent at levels below 1 mmol/L. Although up to a third of patients on long-term lithium therapy develop polyuria, proven morphological changes in the kidney are confined to the distal tubules and collecting ducts, and are reversible. Polyuria is not a reason for discontinuing lithium unless the patient finds it intolerable. Hypothyroidism can be a problem but is not a sufficient reason for discontinuing lithium. Replacement therapy with thyroxine should be commenced.

Toxicity is very likely at concentrations above 1.5 mmol/L. Severe gastrointestinal disturbance, drowsiness, ataxia and dysarthria are early signs of lithium toxicity. If in doubt, lithium should be discontinued until a serum level can be obtained.

Bouts of vomiting, diarrhoea or any form of dehydration will lead to sodium depletion, and, therefore, to increased serum lithium levels. Similarly, a salt-free diet is contraindicated. It is also wise to ensure that the patient is aware of the importance of maintaining an adequate fluid balance (e.g. if working or holidaying in a hot environment).

Carbamazepine

Although used primarily as an anticonvulsant, carbamazepine is sometimes used as a mood stabiliser when response to lithium is inadequate or side effects intolerable. It is possibly more effective than lithium in rapid cycling bipolar disorder (four or more episodes a year). Carbamazepine is associated with rash, leucopenia, hyponatraemia and abnormal liver function tests (LFTs). It is prudent to have baseline values for LFTs, FBC and U&Es available.

It is important to start treatment with a low dose and gradually titrate upwards over a period of two to three weeks: 100–200 mg twice daily would be a reasonable starting dose; at least 300 mg twice daily is required for treatment. Too high a starting dose will lead to problems with ataxia, drowsiness and nausea.

Monitoring the serum concentration is useful to check adherence or suspected toxicity. A minimum level of 8–12 mg/L is usually required for response.

Carbamazepine is a hepatic enzyme inducer, increasing its own metabolism as well as that of several other commonly prescribed drugs. For example, oestrogen-containing oral contraceptives can be rendered ineffective. If these are used concurrently, preparations containing at least 50 µg oestrogen are necessary. Conversely, hepatic enzyme-inhibiting drugs can raise carbamazepine serum levels and so precipitate signs of toxicity. Erythromycin, cimetidine and calcium channel-blocking drugs are commonly prescribed examples.

Other antiepileptic drugs used as mood stabilisers

Valproate is widely used as a mood stabiliser (Box 22.12). It is more effective in preventing manic than depressive episodes. Mild gastrointestinal side effects and weight gain are common. Rarely, valproate can cause thrombocytopenia and hepatic reactions.

Lamotrigine is also used as a mood stabiliser. It is more effective in preventing depressive than manic episodes. The dosage must be titrated up slowly to avoid serious skin reactions, including Stevens–Johnson syndrome. Lamotrigine should only be initiated by specialists; its teratogenicity is less than valproate but it should be used with caution in women of childbearing age.

Clonazepam is a benzodiazepine used occasionally to supplement antiepileptic treatment. As it is a partial agonist at central

---

Box 22.11 Starting and monitoring lithium

Preliminary tests (before starting treatment)
- Renal function tests (urea and electrolytes, U&Es)
- Thyroid function tests (TFTs)
- Full blood count (FBC)
- Blood pressure
- ECG

Starting treatment
- Starting dose of 400 mg/day
- Test blood concentration after seven days
- Titrate oral dose to achieve blood of 0.4–1.0 mmol/L
- Monitor blood concentrations weekly until stable

Monitoring treatment
- Blood sample should be collected 12 hours after last dose
- If on twice-daily regimen, collect blood before morning dose
- Repeat estimates of lithium concentration, TFTs, U&Es, FBC every four to six months during maintenance phase

Drug interactions
- Non-steroidal anti-inflammatory drugs (NSAIDs), ACE inhibitors, angiotensin-2 receptor antagonists and diuretics can all reduce the excretion of lithium resulting in toxicity
- Careful monitoring of plasma levels is required if any of these drugs are started, stopped or the dosage altered

Box 22.12 **Starting and monitoring valproate**

Preliminary tests (before starting treatment)
- Renal function tests (U&Es)
- Full blood count (FBC)

Starting treatment
- Starting dose of 500–750 mg/day
- Titrate oral dose to achieve blood concentration of 50–100 mg/L

Monitoring treatment
- Trough blood sample is required for serum level
- FBC & LFTs repeated every six months during maintenance phase

Women of childbearing age
- Valproate is very teratogenic; the risk of major malformation is increased several-fold over background rates. The strongest association is with neural tube defects
- If there is no alternative to valproate, women should use adequate contraception or prophylactic folate be given

GABA receptors, it may be less liable to cause dependence than other benzodiazepines. It has a specialist role in short-term control of sleep disturbance and agitation in mania.

Concordance with treatment

Agreement with and adherence (compliance) to a treatment regimen is termed concordance. Poor adherence to prescribed treatment is a major problem with almost all psychotropic drugs. Compared with patients who relapse in spite of good adherence, those with poor adherence to treatment are more severely ill at the point of readmission to hospital, have more frequent readmissions, are more likely to be admitted compulsorily and have longer inpatient stays. Adherence itself has a protective effect distinct from the pharmacological benefits of the medication.

Common law: in an emergency, treatment can be given under the common law principles of duty of care and doctrine of necessity

Reasons for failing to achieve concordance involve problems with comprehension, comfort and collaboration.

Comprehension: problems include difficulties in appraising the importance of taking drugs. Patients and their families often have an inadequate understanding of the advantages and limitations of medication.

Comfort: this refers to unpleasant aspects of the treatment such as side effects. Patients with schizophrenia are highly likely to identify parkinsonian side effects as the reason for poor adherence, and non-adherers are less likely to have been prescribed antiparkinsonian medication. Dysphoria, sedation, weight gain, sexual disturbances and galactorrhoea in female patients, are other side effects of drugs that contribute to poor adherence. The side effects are usually experienced before any therapeutic effect, both with antipsychotic and antidepressant medication.

Box 22.13 **Collaborating with patients in drug choice**

This is central to all NICE guidance
- The patient has a right to be consulted about their drug treatment
- They must be given information that is factually accurate and true
- Information should be appropriately presented (in a way that the patient can understand)

Box 22.14 **Strategies to improve concordance with drug treatment**

- When starting treatment, explain the time course of effects. Patients need to be aware that any therapeutic effect may take weeks while side effects will be noticeable immediately. This should be emphasised again at follow-up appointments
- Identify and treat side effects promptly. Prophylactic antiparkinsonian treatment is useful for some patients taking antipsychotic drugs
- Be realistic about what the drug can and cannot do. Many patients have highly unrealistic expectations of benefits
- When possible, start with a low dose and increase it gradually: this reduces the incidence of side effects
- Use minimum dose necessary to achieve desired therapeutic effects
- Use for an adequate period of time
- Use patient information leaflets to provide a written back-up of verbal information
- Involve patients in monitoring their own treatment

Consent should be seen as a process and not as a single event. Patients are able to change their mind and can withdraw consent at any stage

Collaboration: poor adherence can also be viewed as a result of a breakdown in the collaboration between patient and doctor (Box 22.13). It has been argued that schizophrenic patients, particularly young people and those from ethnic minorities, perceive psychiatric treatment as coercive and disempowering. Promising results have been obtained with programmes that combine giving information with efforts to encourage schizophrenic patients to collaborate with professionals in monitoring their treatment (Box 22.14).

Further information

- Contact your local mental health trust pharmacy to find a pharmacist who specialises in psychotropic medication
- In the United Kingdom and the Republic of Ireland, information may be obtained by telephoning regional drug information services or poisons information centres. An up to date list of telephone numbers is given in the current *British National Formulary*

- Rethink (formerly the National Schizophrenia Fellowship), the Royal College of Psychiatrists, and the United Kingdom Psychiatric Pharmacy Group (UKPPG), produce clear and informative leaflets for patients
- Clozapine manufacturers provide information about all aspects of clozapine treatment to doctors who are registered with the service

Further reading

Davies T. Consent to treatment. *Psych Bull* 1997; **21:** 200–1.

National Institute for Health and Clinical Excellence. *Guidance on the use of newer (atypical) antipsychotics in the treatment of schizophrenia.* NICE, London, 2002. www.nice.org.uk

National Institute for Health and Clinical Excellence. *Schizophrenia: Core interventions in the treatment and management of schizophrenia in primary and secondary care.* NICE guideline CG1. NICE, London, 2002. http://guidance.nice.org.uk/CG1/

National Institute for Health and Clinical Excellence. *Guidance on the use of zaleplon, zolpidem and zopiclone for the short-term management of insomnia.* NICE, London, 2004. www.nice.org.uk.

National Institute for Health and Clinical Excellence. *Newer drugs for epilepsy in adults.* NICE technology appraisal guidance 76. NICE, London, 2004. http://guidance.nice.org.uk/TA76/

National Institute for Health and Clinical Excellence. *Bipolar disorder: The management of bipolar disorder in adults, children and adolescents, in primary and secondary care.* NICE guideline CG38. NICE, London, 2006. http://guidance.nice.org.uk/CG38/

National Institute for Health and Clinical Excellence. *Anxiety (amended): Management of anxiety (panic disorder, with or without agoraphobia, and generalised anxiety disorder) in adults in primary, secondary and community care.* NICE guideline CG22. NICE, London, 2007. http://guidance.nice.org.uk/CG22/

National Institute for Health and Clinical Excellence. *Depression (amended): Management of depression in primary and secondary care.* NICE guideline CG23. NICE, London, 2007. http://guidance.nice.org.uk/CG23/

Royal College of Psychiatrists. *Revised consensus statement on the use of high dose antipsychotic drugs.* Royal College of Psychiatrists, London, 2005. www.rcpsych.org.uk

Taylor D, Paton C, Kerwin R. *The Maudsley prescribing guidelines*, 8th edn. Taylor & Francis, London, 2005.

CHAPTER 23

Psychological Treatments

Suzanne Jolley and Phil Richardson

OVERVIEW

- National Institute for Health and Clinical Excellence (NICE) guidance recommends psychological intervention for many mental health problems, but availability of psychological treatment is variable

- Cognitive behavioural therapy (CBT) is an overall term for therapies that utilise behaviour therapy, behaviour modification and cognitive therapy; it is indicated for anxiety disorders, moderate depression and positive features of schizophrenia

- Dialectical behaviour therapy (DBT) may enable people with borderline personality disorder to recognise and manage their unstable emotions

- Psychodynamic psychotherapies aim at resolving the unconscious conflicts that are thought to underlie symptoms; it is used to treat neuroses (anxiety-based disorders) and personality disorders

- Counselling is recommended by NICE as a primary care treatment for mild (but not moderate or severe) depression; it may help people without diagnosable mental disorders to deal with transient life crises

---

The range of procedures that pass for psychological treatment is broad. Over 450 distinct forms of psychotherapy have been identified, although many can be reduced to a narrower set of therapy types. The great diversity of psychological treatments is potentially a source of confusion for referrers, patients and purchasers. Variation in training and accreditation processes can also generate confusion.

The majority of formal psychological therapy in mental health services in the NHS (Box 23.1) is delivered by qualified clinical and counselling psychologists, who are usually regulated through the chartership procedures of the British Psychological Society. However, the delivery of psychological therapy is not limited to psychologists; other mental health professionals often undertake training in psychological therapies, and it is common to be accredited as a practitioner of psychological therapy without a professional mental health qualification. Several professional and regulatory organisations exist, and registration of therapists has been on a voluntary basis with no single professional accreditation

ABC of Mental Health, 2nd edition. Edited by T. Davies and T. Craig.
© 2009 Blackwell Publishing, ISBN: 978-0-7279-1639-6.

Box 23.1 **Psychological treatments most commonly available in the NHS**

- Cognitive behavioural therapy
- Psychodynamic psychotherapy
- Family work (systemic or cognitive behavioural)
- Group therapy
- Various forms of counselling
- Eclectic and integrative approaches

body. In an effort to address this, the UK Department of Health is devising procedures for the statutory registration of psychologists, with other psychological therapists likely to be considered in the future.

Establishment of the National Institute for Health and Clinical Excellence (NICE) and the publication of its treatment guidelines has clarified the choice of therapy to some degree. Guidelines are based on detailed reviews of the evidence for a range of treatments, and psychological intervention – particularly cognitive behavioural therapy (CBT) – is recommended for many mental health problems.

However, the recommendations have not resulted in increased access or availability. Services, and pathways to therapy, vary locally, but overall the increased potential demand has served to highlight the lack of adequate therapy resources in the NHS. Further, NICE offers little in the way of defining either the therapies or those who have the competence to deliver them, thus some confusion around standards remains. The Department of Health Improving Access to Psychological Therapies (IAPT) funds new accredited training programmes, particularly in CBT for anxiety and depression, to train more practitioners to achieve specified competences.

Cognitive behavioural therapy

The term CBT refers to a group of therapies that includes behaviour therapy, behaviour modification and cognitive therapy in various combinations. More recently, 'mindfulness' and acceptance-based approaches or 'third wave' CBT interventions have been developed and are starting to be evaluated. Computerised CBT packages have also been developed, and two of these are recommended by NICE for the treatment of less severe anxiety and depression.

All cognitive behavioural approaches are based on the principle of learning particular patterns of responses (cognitive or behavioural)

Box 23.2 Cognitive behavioural therapy (CBT)

Principles
- Based on learning theory and incorporating both behavioural and cognitive interventions
- Structured and collaborative
- Goal-directed rather than primarily exploratory
- Uses formal techniques for behavioural or cognitive change
- Focused on enabling patients to think, feel and act differently
- Aims for change lasting beyond the end of therapy

Treatment
- Individual or group
- Inpatient or outpatient
- Typically offered on an individual outpatient basis for a time-limited course
- Short term or longer term
- Also recommended as a computer-aided package

Box 23.3 Common problems for which CBT is recommended

Evidence base for CBT for a range of disorders is strong
- Anxiety disorders (panic, specific phobias, social phobia, post-traumatic stress disorder, generalised anxiety disorder, obsessions and compulsions)
- Depression
- Psychosis: especially persisting positive symptoms

Box 23.4 Psychodynamic psychotherapy

Psychotherapeutic techniques
- Exploratory
- Based on psychoanalytic theory, the distinctive feature of which is the focus on resolution of unconscious conflicts

Treatment
- Makes direct use of transference (the patient's experience of the therapist and therapeutic relationship)
- Aims to promote greater conscious understanding of difficulties by the patient, and to enable assimilation of potentially painful and previously avoided experience
- Traditionally long term, but brief variants also available
- Lack of large-scale systematic research means evidence base is currently limited, therefore refer on the basis of client preference

---

through experience, and the primary approach to change involves revaluating this learning and developing new patterns (Box 23.2).

Behavioural approaches draw on the principles of Pavlovian 'classical' conditioning (systematic desensitisation, aversion therapy), Skinnerian operant conditioning (contingency management, activity scheduling) or social learning theory (participant modelling). Formal behavioural analysis of a patient's problem (Box 23.3) is typically followed by individually tailored application of techniques to change behaviour. Change in behaviour is viewed as paramount, both as a therapeutic aim in its own right and in mediating other symptomatic improvement.

Cognitive approaches emphasise how thoughts and other cognitive events (e.g. images) influence feelings and behaviour. They aim to modify thought processes directly. Therapy consists of working with patients to identify unhelpful and often automatic thought patterns (such as hopelessness in depression) and learning to recognise and change these.

'Third wave' approaches aim to facilitate a change in the person's relationship with his or her cognitions, rather than a content change, to allow the recognition of thoughts and other mental events as passing phenomena, which do not necessarily require active consideration. Attention training and meditation techniques are often used to achieve this change. This 'distancing' approach is often combined with more standard cognitive or behavioural interventions. Changing relationships with thoughts is combined with promotion of active engagement in valued activities and behaviours in acceptance and commitment therapy (ACT).

The addition of mindfulness techniques to CBT for depression appears to help reduce relapse.

Dialectical behaviour therapy (DBT) draws on mindfulness techniques combined with cognitive and behavioural strategies to enable people with borderline personality disorders to recognise and manage volatile affect. Although these approaches are relatively new, evidence for their effectiveness is accumulating, and mindfulness-based CBT is now recommended by NICE as a treatment for recurrent depression.

Psychodynamic therapy

Psychodynamic approaches aim to go beyond symptomatic change by resolving the unconscious conflicts that are thought to underlie symptoms. Long-term psychodynamic psychotherapy may last several years and seeks to achieve a fundamental change in personality (Box 23.4). Its availability on the NHS is limited: few services can offer it on an inpatient basis, though several retain some scope for outpatient work.

Brief psychotherapy typically lasts for six months, with weekly or twice-weekly sessions. Therapeutic work is focused on specific issues in the expectation that improved understanding will enable patients to arrive at more lasting symptomatic change through a process that may extend beyond the end of the treatment.

There has been a growing *rapprochement* in recent years between psychodynamic and cognitive perspectives. For example, a number of psychoanalytic concepts have been recast within a cognitive framework, but the therapeutic focus on the resolution of unconscious conflict remains a distinctive feature. There have been very few randomised controlled trials of psychodynamic psychotherapy for any disorder, and thus its effectiveness in treating many difficulties is uncertain.

Counselling

There is no universally agreed definition of counselling, and limited consensus over the distinction between counselling and psychotherapy. In practice, counselling is commonly practised in primary care and the voluntary sector, usually on a short-term basis

(4–10 sessions) by individuals who are not from the core mental health professions but generally have a formal qualification in counselling itself.

A broad distinction can be made between methods based on a specific theoretical framework (such as psychodynamic counselling) or targeting a particular problem (as in bereavement counselling), and generic counselling, which draws on a range of general interpersonal skills (such as reflective listening) and, in the UK, is commonly built on a humanistic or client-centred foundation. Counselling is often used to help people cope better with non-clinical distress associated with immediate crises, to understand better their reactions to events, and to make decisions more effectively about important issues (Box 23.5). It is recommended by NICE as a primary care treatment for mild (but not moderate or severe) depression, but it is unlikely to be a useful first-line intervention with more complex and severe mental health problems reaching diagnostic criteria, although it can be offered as an adjunctive treatment.

Eclectic and integrative approaches

Although there is an increasing emphasis in the NHS on delivering evidence-based interventions, often meaning prioritisation of cognitive behavioural interventions, many practitioners of psychological treatments draw on the principles of various therapeutic approaches while working with an individual patient. Depending on the identified foci for intervention, several different methods may be combined in the course of treatment. This eclectic approach has the advantage of flexibility, but it is difficult to evaluate as its nature changes from case to case and therapist to therapist.

Integrative approaches to therapy also combine the precepts and practices of different therapeutic methods, but in a way that recombines the elements to form a new coherent structure. In Britain, cognitive analytic therapy (CAT) is a popular form of brief integrative therapy that builds on the elements of both CBT and psychodynamic approaches.

Family approaches

Traditional family therapy exemplifies the 'systemic' approach to understanding and modifying problematic behaviour and experience. The family (or other social system), rather than the individual patient, becomes the focus of understanding and intervention. A patient's problem is seen as serving a strategic function

in maintaining some aspect of the family's functioning. The therapist's task is to identify this function and help the family move towards a more adaptive mode of operation.

Family therapists may use direct behavioural modification of a symptom, not as a therapeutic end in itself but as a means to identify the dysfunctional family system. Modifying the system itself may also be achieved through the planned application of various specific technical manoeuvres (such as positive reframing of the symptom, symptom prescription and paradoxical injunction).

In principle, systemic approaches to therapy make no prior assumption about the membership of the social group at which the intervention is targeted. 'Adult' families, partial families and other social groups are equally eligible for systems-based work. Family therapy is often available in the Child and Adolescent Mental Health Services (CAMHS), where a child presents initially as the patient but is viewed as the vehicle of expression of a dysfunctional family system. There is evidence for recommending this approach in eating disorders (especially in younger anorexic patients) and psychophysiological disorders.

Family therapy is distinct from family intervention (FI; Box 23.6) approaches developed specifically for families with a member affected by schizophrenia spectrum psychosis, from cognitive behavioural couple or marital therapy and from behavioural work with families in CAMHS. These approaches, although informed by systemic thinking, tend to focus on developing a shared psychological understanding of the key difficulties; recognising, normalising and working with the emotional reactions of the family/partner and identified patient; and practical and behavioural problem-solving around current difficulties.

Group therapy

Group therapy is a portmanteau term for a wide range of therapeutic approaches in which several patients come together for therapy at the same time and place with one or more therapists. Therapeutic groups may be run according to the principles of any theoretical approach (e.g. CBT, psychodynamic therapy); they may be open (in which new members can join the group after its inception) or closed; inpatient or outpatient; time-limited or open-ended. Their focus may be highly specific (anxiety management groups) or very broad (psychoanalytic group psychotherapy).

Although the economic advantages of therapeutic groups are self-evident, group therapy is not a collective or diluted form of individual therapy. Virtually all group therapies draw on the idea that group processes themselves may be therapeutic. Whenever individual psychotherapy is being considered then it may also be worth considering referral for group therapy. However, assessment for inclusion in a group must take account of the specific group's characteristics, and of the patient's preference for individual therapy or aversion to a group.

Choice of therapeutic method

NICE offers guidance on referral for psychological intervention on a disorder-specific basis according to the current evidence base, and will indicate for most people at least what to attempt first, which is in most cases a cognitive behavioural intervention. The IAPT programme outlines 'low- and high-intensity' interventions for depression and anxiety, whereby brief therapy, guided self-help and computerised therapy are recommended for milder and less complex presentations, with formal therapy delivered by a highly trained practitioner recommended for more complex or severe difficulties.

However, presenting psychological problems do not always fall into neat packages – many do not come within the sphere of diagnosable mental disorder. In these cases, choice of treatment requires assessment of factors that bear on the probable success of a particular treatment for a particular patient, including patient preference (Box 23.7). Decisions should be informed by the evidence base, but for some difficulties the available evidence may be insufficient to the task (Box 23.8). In such cases,

initial referral should be to a coordinated psychological treatments service with expertise in assessment and access to a range of specific therapies, including specialist clinics (such as for psychosexual problems).

Acknowledgment

This chapter is dedicated to the memory of Professor Phil Richardson who died in December 2007.

Box 23.7 Factors affecting choice of psychotherapeutic method

- Nature of problem: diagnosable mental health problem or 'life stress'
- Chronicity: acute, transient or of long standing
- Severity: mild, moderate or severe
- Involvement of family or partner
- Patient preference (although patient should always be advised of evidence-based recommendations)

Box 23.8 Problems in evaluating the psychotherapies

- Relative shortage of controlled trials examining the efficacy of psychodynamic therapies
- Evidence that reaches the highest standards of methodological rigour (from well-conducted randomised controlled trials) is least typical of ordinary clinical practice, where the conditions of the controlled trial are least likely to apply
- Treatment trials and reviews are commonly organised around problem domains (anxiety, depression, etc.), and tell us about the aggregate progress of a group of treated patients compared with that of an untreated group, rather than the impact on particular individuals

---

Further information

- Most providers of psychological therapies within NHS mental health services operate within community mental health teams or within associated specialised psychological, counselling and psychotherapy services
- Psychological therapies, particularly counselling, are often available in primary care
- The regulatory bodies listed below hold databases of registered therapists
- Self-help groups and voluntary organisations are also available in many areas: local libraries often stock self-help manuals, relaxation tapes and other helpful material as well as lists of local voluntary services
- Computerised CBT self-help material is becoming increasingly available and early evaluations suggest it can be effective for mild and less complicated difficulties (see BABCP and NICE websites for details)
- Psychological therapies can also be offered to couples and families, both within the NHS and through organisations such as RELATE
- *Contact: A directory for mental health 2005* lists a wide range of organisations offering help for people with mental health problems: http://www.dh.gov. uk/en/Publicationsandstatistics/Publications/ PublicationsPolicyAndGuidance/DH_4108807
- National Collaborating Centre for Mental Health (NCCMH), established by NICE, is a partnership between the Royal College of Psychiatrists Research and Training Unit (CRTU) and the British Psychological Society Centre for Outcomes Research and Effectiveness (CORE). It is responsible for developing NICE mental health guidelines: www.nccmh.org.uk; www.nice. org.uk; www.rcpsych.ac.uk/crtu.aspx; www.ucl.ac.uk/ clinical-psychology/CORE
- Department of Health – Mental Health Publications – Improving Access to Psychological Therapies: various guidance documents, www.dh.gov.uk
- MIND: a range of leaflets on therapies and mental health problems, www.mind.org.uk
- Sainsbury Centre for Mental Health: information leaflets on talking therapies, www.scmh.org.uk
- Royal College of Psychiatrists: leaflets on therapies and mental health problems, www.rcpsych.ac.uk
- Mental Health Foundation: a charity campaigning on mental health issues and with many leaflets about mental health problems and therapies, www.mentalhealth.org.uk

Main organisations accrediting and regulating psychotherapists in the UK
- United Kingdom Council for Psychotherapy (UKCP): umbrella organisation for the regulation and promotion of psychotherapy, www.psychotherapy.org.uk
- British Psychoanalytic Council (BPC): umbrella regulatory organisation for psychotherapists and smaller psychotherapy organisations, www.psychoanalytic-council.org
- British Association of Psychotherapists (BAP): offers therapy and associated resources including information and training, www.bap-psychotherapy.org
- British Association for Counselling and Psychotherapy (BACP): regulatory and accrediting body for individuals and training courses; provides information and lists of accredited therapists, www.bacp.co.uk
- British Psychological Society (BPS): regulatory professional association for academic, clinical and other chartered psychologists, www.bps.org.uk
- British Association for Behavioural and Cognitive Psychotherapies (BABCP): accrediting and regulatory body for CBT and behavioural therapy; provides useful information on therapy and training, www.babcp.com
- Health Professions Council (HPC): the body identified by the government through which psychological therapy providers are likely to be regulated on a statutory basis, www.hpc-uk.org

Further reading

Department of Health. *Choosing talking therapies. Treatment choice in psychological therapies and counselling: Evidence based clinical practice guideline.* DH, London, 2001.

Feltham C, Horton I (eds). *The SAGE handbook of counselling and psychotherapy*, 2nd edn. SAGE Publications, London, 2006.

Hawton K, Salkovskis PM, Kirk J, Clark DM. *Cognitive behaviour therapy for psychiatric problems: A practical guide.* Oxford University Press, Oxford, 1998.

Hayes SC, Strosahl KD (eds). *A practical guide to acceptance and commitment therapy.* Springer, New York, 2004.

Kuipers L, Leff JP, Lam D. *Family work for schizophrenia: A practical guide*, 2nd edn. Gaskell, London, 2005.

Linehan MM. *Cognitive–behavioral treatment of borderline personality disorder.* Guilford Press, New York, 1993.

Mace C. Mindfulness in psychotherapy: an introduction. *Adv Psych Treatment* 2007; **13:** 147–54.

Miller WR, Rollnick S. *Motivational interviewing: Preparing people for change*, 2nd edn. Guilford Press, New York, 2002.

National Institute for Health and Clinical Excellence. *Schizophrenia: Core interventions in the treatment and management of schizophrenia in primary and secondary care.* NICE guideline CG1. NICE, London, 2002. http://guidance.nice.org.uk/CG1/

National Institute for Health and Clinical Excellence. *Computerised cognitive behaviour therapy for depression and anxiety. Review of Technology Appraisal 51.* NICE technology appraisal 97 guidance. NICE, London, 2006. http://www.nice.org.uk/nicemedia/pdf/TA097guidance.pdf

National Institute for Health and Clinical Excellence. *Anxiety (amended): Management of anxiety (panic disorder, with or without agoraphobia, and generalised anxiety disorder) in adults in primary, secondary and community care.* NICE guideline CG22. NICE, London, 2007. http://guidance.nice.org.uk/CG22/

National Institute for Health and Clinical Excellence. *Depression (amended): Management of depression in primary and secondary care.* NICE guideline CG23. NICE, London, 2007. http://guidance.nice.org.uk/CG23/

Pilling S, Bebbington P, Kuipers E, *et al.* Psychological treatments in schizophrenia. I: Meta-analysis of family intervention and CBT. *Psychol Med* 2002; **32:** 763–82.

Roth A, Fonagy P. *What works for whom? A critical review of psychotherapy research*, 2nd edn. Guilford Press, New York, 2004.

Segal Z, Teasdale J, Williams M. *Mindfulness-based cognitive therapy for depression.* Guilford Press, New York, 2002.

CHAPTER 24

Risk Management in Mental Health

Teifion Davies

OVERVIEW

- Risk is the probability of occurrence of an event, regardless of whether the event is wanted or unwanted

- All clinical actions carry risk of harmful events, and assessment of these risks is intrinsic to clinical decision-making; in mental health, harmful outcomes include side effects of treatment, suicide and violence

- Several instruments exist to estimate a patient's risk of violent behaviour; most are based on data from populations with high prevalence of such behaviour, and are not applicable to community or general inpatient settings

- Assessment of immediate and short-term risks depends mainly on the patient's clinical state, while medium and longer term risks may be predicted from the patient's demographic characteristics

- Several risk factors for suicide or violence are recognised, but predictive value of individual factors is seriously limited

Risks and uncertainties abound in all branches of medicine, and assessing risk has always been an important aspect of clinical work. This is not confined to psychiatry: any patient may, as a consequence of an illness or its treatment, be exposed to risk or pose a risk to other people.

However, a formal assessment of risks to patients (due to their illness or its treatment) or to other people (due to violence or neglect by a patient) is seen increasingly as a routine component of management of mental health problems, and an essential component of a patient's care plan under the care programme approach. Previous chapters have dealt with the major risks associated with specific mental health problems. This chapter draws together the common features of clinical risk management in mental health.

General principles

Strictly speaking, a risk is the probability of an event occurring, where the event may be desirable (such as recovery from illness) or undesirable (such as side effects of drug treatment, relapse, suicide or harm to others). Risk management has three principal components: identification, analysis and control.

ABC of Mental Health, 2nd edition. Edited by T. Davies and T. Craig.
© 2009 Blackwell Publishing, ISBN: 978-0-7279-1639-6.

Identification

The essential first stage, which may seem obvious, is recognising that risks may arise from all aspects of clinical work and provision of healthcare. Factors as diverse as the layout of a surgery or ward, staffing levels and training, design of documents and records, and means of communication between services and prescribing practices may raise or lower risks. These 'background' factors apply to all patients and clinical situations, but the need to be aware of them extends well beyond the doctors and nurses on the front line.

Specific risks associated with particular clinical situations or groups of patients should be identified. This will include the type and frequency of risks, the circumstances in which they arise and the people subject to them. In any healthcare organisation (such as hospital or general practice surgery), identification will depend on well-developed programmes of audit and quality assurance, the prevalent 'culture' and attitudes, and available knowledge.

Analysis

Risk is an actuarial concept, and analysis depends on quantifying several variables – risk factors – and their interactions. Although some risk factors (such as a patient's personality) may remain constant over long periods, others will be variable (for instance, with changes in mental state or environment). So, the estimated probability of occurrence will vary with time, and range from zero (no chance of the event occurring) to one (complete certainty that the event will occur).

The tests used to quantify a particular risk will be subject to the same constraints of sensitivity and specificity, and of errors of estimation, that apply to any measurement technique.

Control

Control of risk depends on the type of risk identified, its estimated size and the resources available. Formal programmes for risk management in healthcare organisations emphasise economic aspects: weighing the resources needed to control risks against the anticipated costs of untoward events. 'Costs' include effects on staff morale and damage to the organisation's reputation, as well as more obvious clinical and legal costs.

Staff should be aware of the likely risks in their sphere of practice and of the risk-management strategies. As 'risk' implies uncertainty, there should be a culture of 'expecting the unexpected', and of knowing what to do if the unexpected occurs. This will include

Box 24.1 **Clinical risks and clinical decision-making**

- All clinical decisions carry risks, and all clinical decision-making should be seen as part of risk management
- Decisions may concern type of diagnosis, choice of treatment, need for admission to hospital, or fitness for discharge from hospital. In mental health, decisions may also concern compulsory admission and treatment and safety of other people
- Decisions often involve a choice between several options, each of which has its associated risks
- Decisions may involve comparing different risks (treating a patient with antipsychotic drugs may cause severe side effects, whereas not treating the patient may risk violence to others)
- None of the available options may be clearly superior to all the others
- Whenever possible, options should be discussed in a multidisciplinary context
- The reasons for choosing a particular option should be stated clearly in the care plan, including
  - Which options were considered
  - What information was available
  - The perceived risks of each option
  - What changes in circumstances would prompt a review of the decision

A date should be set to review risk assessment and care plan

a rapid response to untoward events, caring for victims (patients, staff and others) and recording information.

Recent inquiries have pointed to the need to warn potential victims of important risks, to take account of their fears and plan for their safety (Box 24.1).

Clinical risk

Clinical risk concerns the potential for harm posed by, or inflicted on, an individual patient. The risk of a clinically important event occurring is best regarded as ranging from low (very unlikely) to high (very likely). This restricted range of probabilities takes account of the difficulties in applying actuarial data derived from populations to individual clinical situations.

Clinical risk factors divide roughly into two types: demographic and patient factors. Demographic factors relate to the risks in populations of patients, and tend to be relatively fixed or slowly evolving in time; they comprise the baseline level of risk in that population, but have poor temporal resolution. Patient risk factors form a pattern that is specific to a particular patient: they may be highly variable in time, so requiring repeated monitoring rather than one-off assessment.

In mental health the risks of greatest concern are suicide, self-harm, violence to others and neglect of dependents. Other risks are those familiar in all branches of medicine: morbidity and cumulative disability from illness, side effects of medical treatment (such as drugs or electroconvulsive therapy) and untoward outcomes of other treatments (including psychotherapy and complementary therapies).

Risk-assessment instruments

A number of scales and instruments exist to assist in formalising assessment of clinical risk, most often risk of violent behaviour. These attempt to combine actuarial data from populations with clinical information pertaining to the individual patient. Amongst the most widely adopted is the HCR-20, a 20-item scale that links historical, clinical and specific risk information to predict a patient's future propensity to violence.

Predictive value of a diagnostic test depends on the prevalence of the condition in the population. As the prevalence falls, 'positive' test results are increasingly likely to be false

Although these techniques improve on simple clinical judgement, especially in the long term, their predictive value in individual cases is limited as they are based on factors derived from very high-risk populations (forensic cases or prison inmates). Even when applied to patients such as those on which they are based, they achieve only about 70% accuracy in the longer term. They are also time-consuming to compile, provide little guidance on short- or medium-term risks and are of little help in the acute clinical situation.

Practical aspects of clinical risk assessment

The reliability of a clinical risk assessment is greatest at the time it is performed and declines rapidly afterwards. For this reason, each risk should be dealt with separately, its timescale (immediate, short term, medium term or long term) delineated and a time set for a further assessment to be made. A full risk assessment will require attention to each of these time periods, and of their interplay with the patient's diagnosis and treatment (Box 24.2). Assessing immediate and short-term risks relies heavily on clinical (i.e. patient) factors, whereas assessing medium and longer term risks is informed by stable, demographic data based on populations of patients.

Immediate risks

These require immediate action to avoid an untoward event. They may arise from a sudden crisis in a patient's life or from fluctuations in his or her mental state. Assessment should focus on the patient's observed behaviour, level of emotional arousal, expression of intentions or threats and psychomotor agitation, supplemented by as full an examination of the mental state as is practicable.

Short-term risks

These are predictable over the next few hours or days. Assessment requires a knowledge of the patient's insight, coping mechanisms and level of support, as well as an evaluation of ongoing crises and their potential resolution.

Box 24.2 **Practical steps in managing a patient's risk**

Even in a crisis, an attempt should be made to perform the following steps as fully as possible:

- **Accumulate information from clinical and non-clinical sources:** including the current mental state and response to treatment. Include eye witness accounts, and details from family and neighbours where necessary
- **Identify gaps and discrepancies in the history:** are there periods during which the patient lost contact with services? If so, attempt to obtain missing information
- **Construct a chronological listing of significant events in patient's life:** include episodes of violence or suicidal behaviour, episodes of illness, treatment and response
- **Identify patterns of behaviour:** is risk-taking haphazard, associated with specific circumstances (such as relapse of illness, social upheavals, drug or alcohol misuse) or particular people (such as family, neighbours, passers-by in the street)?
- **Assess risk of similar events recurring:** will the patient be exposed to similar situations in the future? If so, what can be done to minimise risk of harm occurring?
- **Disseminate information to all involved in the patient's care:** all members of the clinical team should be aware of signs of relapse, or of impending violent or suicidal behaviour. The general practitioner should be included at all stages of discussion
- **Discuss the risks with the patient and his or her carers:** outline the perceived risks and the care plan. Indicate clearly whom to contact in an emergency. Respect confidentiality, but avoid being drawn into collusion or 'keeping secrets'. Make it clear that, in the interests of safety, information should be shared on a 'need to know' basis
- **Treat mental disorder:** always prescribe adequate drug treatment, and appropriate psychological interventions, as indicated. Where there is a risk that drugs will be misused, arrangements should be made for safe storage and administration
- **Keep clear clinical records:** this will facilitate the task of future risk assessment
- **Review the risk assessment and care plan:** the value of an isolated assessment diminishes rapidly, and depends on changes in a patient's mental state and circumstances. Reviews should be scheduled at regular intervals, e.g. hourly in a crisis. Any important changes should trigger earlier review

Medium-term risks

These are risks expected during the current episode of illness. The patient's provisional diagnosis and likely adherence and expected response to treatment are important in predicting risks during the current episode. The presence of specific risk factors (such as depressive, persecutory and emotional phenomena) should be allowed for in the care plan.

Long-term risks

These are the 'baseline' risks that a patient exhibits between acute episodes of illness, which may remain reasonably constant or evolve gradually over many years. They are influenced by demographic factors such as the patient's age, sex and social class. For a specific patient, these will be modified by diagnosis, enduring personality factors (such as emotional instability, poor coping and low tolerance of frustration), social circumstances and patterns of behaviour (such as remorse, help-seeking, alcohol and drug misuse, and adherence to treatment).

Sources of information

In assessments of immediate and short-term risks, the patient's observed behaviour and his or her mental state provide most information. In order to assess longer term risks and place short-term risks in context, as much collateral information as possible should be sought. This will include general practice records and medical and psychiatric case notes, and may require tracing contacts with services in other districts. In some cases, police or probation service records and local newspaper reports may provide further information.

Personal accounts from family, friends, neighbours or healthcare staff may be particularly important for providing details of unrecorded incidents of dangerous or self-harming behaviour. It is worth remembering that these people may be the ones most at risk from a potentially violent patient (Box 24.3).

Interviews, handled sensitively, may serve the dual purpose of gaining information and informing potential victims of risks and contingency plans.

In practice, it is easiest to build up a picture of the risks posed by an individual patient (Box 24.4) if the clinical case notes provide a simple chronological record. It is important to remember that the structure of case notes should always be subservient to the function of clinical risk management.

Box 24.3 **Risk of violent behaviour associated with acute psychotic disorder**

Mr C, a 22-year-old student at a teacher-training college, became increasingly withdrawn and isolated, spending several days alone in his room at a hall of residence. He consulted the student health physician with complaints that 'something was going on' and his mind was being read by the students living on the floor above his room. He was prescribed antipsychotic drugs, and referred to the local psychiatric clinic. He stopped taking his drug treatment after two days because of unacceptable side effects, which he attributed to 'being poisoned'.

A week later, he set a fire in his room in the belief that the smoke would prevent his thoughts being read. Considerable damage was caused, but prompt action by the emergency services prevented loss of life. He was arrested and charged with arson with intent to endanger life. At psychiatric interview, he showed features of paranoid schizophrenia, and the court ordered that he should be detained for treatment under section 37 of the Mental Health Act 1983.

He was treated with gradually increasing doses of antipsychotic drugs, and responded well with few side effects. He returned to his college course after one year, with the knowledge and support of the college authorities.

Suicide

International comparisons suggest that the suicide rate in the UK is falling (currently 8/100,000/year and amongst the lowest in Europe), whereas in countries of the former Soviet Union rates are ten times higher and rising. In the UK, death by suicide is about twice as common in men as women until middle age when the rates are closer. In recent years the rate in young, often unemployed, men has risen by about 75%, and some surveys have noted similar increases in young women. Several demographic factors are associated with raised risk of suicide (Box 24.5), but these have poor sensitivity and specificity when applied to individuals. This may be because of the clear interaction between such factors as young age, unemployment, social deprivation, availability of means, and alcohol and drug misuse.

Several mental disorders carry an increased risk of suicide (Box 24.6), the most important being depressive episode (about 30 times the risk in the general population), schizophrenia and alcohol dependence. However, 'neurotic' disorders (such as social phobia and panic attacks) and personality disorders (particularly those with emotional instability or self-harm) also confer an increased risk.

Assessment

In assessing an individual patient's suicide risk, careful evaluation of depressive symptoms (such as hopelessness) – together with direct

inquiry about suicidal thoughts, intentions and plans – is most important. Other critical factors are the nature of the precipitating events, the presence of serious physical illness and the presence of social support (especially personal relationships).

Risks to others, especially dependent or physically ill relatives, should be considered. A patient experiencing nihilistic ideas or overwhelmed by a relative's chronic illness may contrive a 'suicide pact' or mercy killing as part of his or her own suicide plans.

Management

When substantial mental disorder, such as depression, is present, it should be treated adequately: the patient and his or her carers should be advised of potential side effects of drug treatment. With the patient's agreement, a few days' supply of drugs may be dispensed at a time. A specific appointment should be made for follow-up assessment, and the patient and his or her carers should know whom to contact if matters deteriorate further.

Admission to hospital, under the Mental Health Act if necessary, may be the only realistic option. Hospital staff should be aware of the risks posed by a patient, and an appropriate level of vigilance maintained. Discharge plans should involve the carers, and take account of continued suicidal thoughts as other symptoms of depression subside and the patient regains his or her energy.

Violence

The best predictor of violence is a history of violent behaviour (Box 24.7), and many potentially violent patients will have a documented forensic history. Men commit more violent acts than women, often within their family; violence to strangers is rare, and most perpetrators of violence are known to the victim. The predictive value of any single risk factor is limited, and even assessments based on several factors are reliable for only relatively short periods.

Although schizophrenia is the mental disorder most often associated with violence in the public mind, the absolute risk in an individual patient is not high. Some personality disorders (especially those in cluster B – dissocial, impulsive and emotionally unstable types), drug and alcohol misuse, and even depression may increase the risk of violence by a patient. Rarely, a patient with a phobic disorder (especially social phobia) may react aggressively if 'trapped' or confined in a crowded place.

Best evidence suggests that comorbidity for some of these conditions (a psychotic illness, a personality disorder and drug or alcohol misuse) increases the risk of violent behaviour. So, although about 2% of people with no psychiatric disorder, and less than 6% of patients with one diagnosis, pose a risk of violence, the rate in patients with two comorbid conditions rises to 8–18%, and in those with three concurrent diagnoses to 12–24%.

Assessment

As with the assessment of suicide risk, demographic factors associated with violence (Box 24.8) show poor specificity and sensitivity when applied to individual patients. The best predictors derive from a thorough knowledge of a patient's patterns of behaviour, habits, coping strategies and tolerance of frustration, in conjunction with an evaluation of his or her mental state.

Although a personal history of violence is an important indicator of long-term risk, it is the pattern and circumstances of such behaviour that is crucial to estimating risk in the short term. Changes in mental symptoms (such as intensifying persecutory delusions), behaviour (such as defaulting on treatment) or personal circumstances are particularly important (Box 24.9).

Box 24.7 Risk of violent behaviour in a 'medical' patient

Mr A, a 56-year-old married man with a long history of diabetes mellitus, was admitted to a medical ward of the general hospital for investigation of chest pain. He had no history of psychiatric disorder. As his meal was served, he became distressed with incoherent speech, and threw his plate at a nurse. He lost consciousness and collapsed.

Urgent tests showed no cardiac abnormality, but his blood glucose concentration was <1.0 mmol/L. After correction of hypoglycaemia, he recovered consciousness with no recall of the events preceding his collapse. Enquiry revealed that he had behaved similarly on several previous occasions, at home and at work, but the incidents had been regarded as trivial and not recorded.

Box 24.8 Demographic (population-based) factors associated with increased risk of violence

- Male
- Younger age
- History of aggressive or violent behaviour, especially involving weapons
- Personality disorder: especially dissocial or impulsive types, and those involving sadistic fantasies
- 'Psychotic' mental illness: especially schizophrenia, morbid jealousy
- Alcohol or drug misuse
- 'Organic' mental state: delirium, acute intoxication
- Unwillingness to accept treatment, or maintain contact with services

---

Management

Management strategies depend on sharing information and responsibilities for monitoring among the clinical team. Important components are treating mental disorder, minimising the side effects of drugs, encouraging contact with services, assisting the patient in developing alternative coping techniques that avoid violence, and pre-empting situations in which violent behaviour is known to occur (Boxes 24.10 and 24.11). Careful consideration should be given to warning carers of predicted risks and involving them in monitoring the patient's mental state.

Box 24.9 Clinical (patient-based) factors associated with increased risk of violence

- Threats or expressed intentions to harm someone
- Lack of regret or remorse for previous violence
- Delusions of passivity, control, jealousy or of sexual interference
- Delusions focused on particular people, especially if the patient feels threatened
- Hallucinations, especially of commands
- Agitation, which may be worsened by side effects of some drug treatments
- Inability to cope with stress or tolerate frustration, especially if associated with impulsive behaviour

---

Box 24.10 Risk of violent behaviour associated with social phobia

Miss B, a 30-year-old woman with a history of social phobia, became agitated while standing in the checkout queue of a busy supermarket. Her behaviour raised the suspicions of the store detective, who instructed two security guards to block the exit to the store. Her desire to escape became intolerable, and she struck a 10-year-old girl who was standing in front of her in the queue.

She was arrested, but became aggressive and unmanageable when placed in a police van with four police officers. She was taken in handcuffs to the local hospital for assessment, and required tranquillisation to prevent her assaulting staff.

At interview, a clear history was elicited of social phobia associated with intolerable feelings of being trapped. She had no formal forensic history, but recalled damaging a telephone box several years earlier when she felt trapped inside.

Box 24.11 Risk of dangerous behaviour associated with panic

Mr D, an 18-year-old man with no history of psychiatric disorder, was encouraged by his girlfriend to take a ride on a big wheel at a fairground. While the wheel was in motion he experienced mild agitation, but attributed this to excitement. When the wheel stopped with his seat high above the ground, he was overwhelmed with panic and a desire to escape. He attempted to release his safety harness and jump out, and his girlfriend risked being dragged out as she tried to restrain him.

Feelings of panic subsided when the wheel started moving, and dissipated completely when he returned to the ground at the end of the ride. He could recall no similar experiences in the past, and has subsequently avoided great heights.

Conclusion: acceptable and defensible risk-taking

As all clinical decisions involve risks (harms and benefits), attempts to avoid risk-taking would paralyse clinical work. Frameworks exist in both health and social care to support clinicians in making decisions that involve risks. These emphasise the need for clinicians and their managers to define in advance the range of acceptable risks when making difficult decisions on limited information with highly uncertain outcomes within each clinical setting.

The decision-making process then proceeds along the lines given in Box 24.2, above: gathering as much relevant information as possible; making it available to all involved in the decision; holding multiprofessional discussions; recording all options considered, and the reasons for choosing or rejecting a course of action; and sharing information and discussion with the patient and his or her carers. The final, critical, requirement is for clinicians to know that, provided they follow accepted procedures, they will be supported by their organisation if an adverse event occurs.

Further information

Royal College of Psychiatrists leaflets available in several languages:
- Depression
- Forensic psychiatric services
- Personality disorders
- Schizophrenia
- Self-harm

Further reading

Calman KC, Royston GHD. Risk language and dialects. *BMJ* 1997; **315**: 939–42.

Department of Health. *Independence, choice and risk: A guide to best practice in supported decision making*. DH, London, 2007.

Gask L, Morriss R. Assessment and immediate management of people at risk of harming themselves. *Psychiatry* 2006; **5**: 266–70.

Langan J, Lindow V. *Living with risk: Mental health service user involvement in risk assessment and management*. Joseph Rowntree Foundation/The Policy Press, Bristol, 2004.

Large M, Smith G, Swinson N, Shaw J, Nielssen O. Homicide due to mental disorder in England and Wales over 50 years. *Br J Psych* 2008; **193**: 130–3.

Norko MA, Baranoski MV. The prediction of violence; detection of dangerousness. *Brief Treat Crisis Intervention* 2008; **8**: 73–91.

Puri BK, Treasaden IH. *Emergencies in psychiatry*. Oxford University Press, Oxford, 2008.

Rose D, Knight M, Fleischmann P, *et al. Scoping study: Public and media perceptions of risk to general public posed by individuals with mental ill health*. Service-User Research Enterprise (SURE), King's College London Institute of Psychiatry, London, 2007.

Royal College of Psychiatrists. *Rethinking risk to others in mental health services*. College Report CR 150, RCPsych, London, 2008.

Szmukler G. Risk assessment: 'numbers' and 'values'. *Psych Bull* 2003; **27**: 205–7.

Thornicroft G. *Shunned: Discrimination against people with mental illness*. Oxford University Press, Oxford, 2006.

Wintrup A. *Assessing risk of violence in mentally disordered offenders with the HCR-20*. Simon Fraser University, Vancouver, 1996.

Index

Abbreviated Mental Test Score 69
acamprosate 63
access to care 23–7
  ethnic minorities 84
  homelessness 87, 88, 89
  psychological treatments 103
  routes to services 26
accident & emergency departments 15–16
acetaldehyde dehydrogenase 61
acetylcholinesterase inhibitors 69–70
acknowledgement of patient distress 9
acute general hospitals 15–18, 20, 23
acute stress reactions 28
addiction 55–9, 60–63
adherence to treatment 17, 101
adjustment reactions 28
admission to hospital 15–18, 20, 23, 50, 91–3
adolescents 72–5, 93
aftercare, violent incidents 21
aggression 8, 9, 19–22, 109–10, 111–12
  self-harm 1, 15–16, 39, 51, 77
agnosia 69
agoraphobia 29, 30–1, 34
akathisia 99
alcohol-related problems
  addiction 60–3
  diagnostic hierarchies 4
  homelessness 86, 87, 88
  physical illness-associated 16
  prevalence 1
Alzheimer-type dementia 68, 69, 71
American Psychiatric Association 48
amnesia 62, 68
amok 83
amphetamine misuse 56, 57, 58
amylobarbitone 21, 22
anorexia nervosa 1, 74
antianxiety medication 99–100
  see also benzodiazepines; serotonin reuptake
    inhibitors
anticholinergic drugs 99
antidepressant drugs
  childbearing 38
  cultural aspects 84
  depression 96
  maintenance treatment 37
  personality disorders 51
  psychiatric disorder in physically-ill patients 17
  psychotherapy comparison 36
  side effects 97

antipsychotic drugs 97–9
  atypical 98
  depot 45, 98
  personality disorders 51
  schizophrenia 45–6, 97–9, 101
  side effects 45, 101
anxiety
  cognitive models 28, 29
  disorders 28–34
  homelessness 88
  intellectual disability 78, 79
  management 29–30, 31, 32, 33
  obsessive–compulsive disorder 29, 33–4
  older people 65–6
  physically-ill patients 17
  physiological symptoms 65
  prevalence 1
  primary care 11–14
  sexual dysfunction 53
apathy 8
aphasia 69
appearance 3
appropriate behaviour modelling 9
approved clinicians 93
apraxia 68
Asperger syndrome 77
assertive outreach teams 24
assessment see diagnosis and assessment
asylums 23
asylum seekers 86, 87
attention deficit hyperactivity disorder 73–4
attorney, power of 93
atypical antipsychotics 97, 98
AUDIT 61
autism 77

behaviour
  see also cognitive behavioural therapy
  coping strategies 7–8
  dementia 70
  distressed patients 7–10
  externalising disorders in children/
    adolescents 73–4
  intellectual disability 76–7
  mental state examination 3
  modelling appropriate 9
  overshadowing 77
  violence prediction 20
benzodiazepines
  alcohol detoxification 62

anxiety disorders 30
  misuse 56
  older people 66
  prescribing 99, 100–101
  rapid tranquillisation 21, 22
  side effects 99
  withdrawal 58
bereavement 11
beta-blockers 30
bipolar affective disorder 1, 38, 40–43, 79, 100
black and minority ethnic groups 87
bodily distress mannerisms 9
body image disorders 17
brain injury 10
bulimia nervosa 74
buprenorphine 58
buspirone 30

CAGE questionnaire 61
Caldicott Guardians 94, 95
calm manner 9, 21
cannabis 56, 57, 58
capacity 3, 91, 92, 93, 94
carbamazepine 100
cardiovascular assessment 3
Care Programme Approach 24, 80
carer support workers 24
challenging behaviour 7–10, 77
  see also violence
Child and Adolescent Mental Health Services 73,
  74, 105
childbearing 38, 40, 101
children 72–5, 93, 105
chlormethiazole 62
chlorpromazine 97
choice questions 2
chronic conditions 12, 35, 37–8, 41–3
classification
  alcohol-related disorders 62
  bipolar disorder 40
  child/adolescent mental health problems 73
  depression 37
  intellectual disability 78
  late-onset paranoid disorders 66
  mania 47
  personality disorders 48, 49
  primary care problem typologies 12
  sexual dysfunction 52–3
clinical risk 108–13
clinical tests 3, 61, 69, 109

clinic layouts 19
clomipramine 34
clonazepam 100–101
closed/open questions 2, 3
clozapine 97, 98, 102
Clunis, Christopher 24
Cluster A/B/C (DSM-IV) disorders 48–50
cocaine 56, 57, 58
cognitive analytic therapy 105
cognitive behavioural therapy
    anxiety disorders 28, 29, 30, 31, 33, 34
    depression 36
    overview 103–4
    physical illness 17, 18
    schizophrenia 46
cognitive models 28, 29
collaboration with patients 101
collateral patient history 3
combination antipsychotics 99
Committee on Safety of Medicines 71
Common Assessment Framework 72
common law duty of care 91, 92, 93, 101
communication difficulties 77, 84
community
    care 23–4, 25, 26, 46
    detoxification 62
    mental health teams 23, 24, 25, 26, 27, 46
    treatment orders 93
competence 93
compliance 17, 101
compulsory admission/treatment 90, 91
concordance with treatment 17, 101
conduct see behaviour
confidentiality 91, 94
confusion 4
consent to treatment 92–3, 101
coping patterns/strategies 7–8
cost of antidepressants 37
counselling 103, 104–5
County Asylums Act (1845) 24
crisis resolution/home treatment teams 24, 27
crisis responses 19–22, 24, 26–7, 41–2, 92
Crown Courts 93
Croydon Integrated Adult Mental Health
    Service 25, 26
cultural aspects 81–5, 86–90
current problems assessment 2, 3
curses (obeah) 82

Data Protection Act (1998) 94
decision-making 109
delirium 4, 66
delirium tremens 60, 61, 62
delusions
    cultural aspects 82
    definition 4, 45
    medication 97
    older people 66
    violence prediction 20
dementia 68–71
denial 8
dependence 55–9, 60–63
depot antipsychotics 45, 98
depression 35–9
    bipolar disorder 38, 41
    childbearing 38
    children/adolescents 74

cultural aspects 81, 82
electroconvulsive therapy 38
forms/types 35–6, 37, 96–7
homelessness 87, 88
medication 36–7, 65, 96–7
mixed states 41
older people 64–5
physically-ill patients 17
prevalence 1
primary care 11–14
seasonal affective disorder 38
self-harm 15, 39
somatic syndrome 36
suicide 2, 13, 22, 39, 97, 111
detention, compulsory 90, 91
detoxification 61–2
developmental disorders 73, 74
dhat 83
diagnosis and assessment
    bipolar disorder 40–41
    dementia 69
    depression 35, 36
    drug misuse 58
    generalised anxiety disorder 30
    initial psychiatric 1–6
    intellectual disability 77–9
    panic disorder 31
    personality disorders 48, 49–50
    post-traumatic stress disorder 33
    schizophrenia 45
    self-harm, hospital situation 16
    social phobias 32
Diagnostic Criteria for Learning Disabilities 78
diagnostic hierarchy of disorders 4
dialectical behaviour therapy 16, 50, 103, 104
diazepam 21
disability rates 5
distressed patients 7–10, 81–2
disulfiram 62–3
dosages 97, 98, 100
Down syndrome 76, 79
drive, fitness to 5
drug misuse 1, 4, 16, 55–9, 88
drug treatments see medication
dysfunctional coping 7–8
dysthymia 35, 37–8
dystonias 99

early intervention teams 24
eating disorders 17, 74, 78, 79
eclectic approach 105
ecstasy 56, 57, 58
elderly people 64–7
electroconvulsive therapy 38
emergencies 15–16, 19–22, 41–2, 92
emotional distress 7–10, 81–2
empathy 9
engagement 12–13
environmental causes 72
epidemiology
    alcohol-related problems 60–61
    anxiety 1
    childhood problems 72–3
    dementia 68
    depression in older people 64
    homelessness 87–8
    personality disorders 49

psychiatric morbidity 1, 15
psychotic disorders in elderly people 66
self-harm/suicide 1, 2, 22, 111
violence 20, 109–10, 111–12
ethnic aspects 81–5
explanations of illness 82
extrapyramidal side effects 97, 98, 99
eye movement desensitisation reprocessing 33

family 3, 72, 83–4, 93, 105
fixed coping behaviour 7–8
FP10 (MDA) prescriptions 58
fragile X syndrome 76
functional aspects 4, 7, 78

gateway primary-secondary workers 25
gender problems 54
generalised anxiety disorder 28–30
general practitioners 11–14, 24–5, 72, 74
genetic predisposition 40, 44, 49
goals, achievable for patients 10
graduate primary care workers 25
grief and loss 11
group therapy 51, 105–6

hallucinations 97
    cultural aspects 82
    definition 4
    older people 66
    schizophrenia 44–5
    violence prediction 20
haloperidol 21, 22
HCR-20 scale 109
healers, traditional 83, 84
The Health of the Nation 60
hepatic enzymes 100
heroin 56, 58
history of service provision 23–4
history-taking, initial 2
homelessness 86–90
hospital admission 15–18
    compulsory 91
    emergency 20
    mental hospitals 23
    mentally disordered offenders 93
    personality disorders 50
    somatisation 17, 18
housing 86–90
Human Rights Act (1998) 91, 92, 94
5-hydroxytryptamine see serotonin reuptake
    inhibitors
hyperkinetic disorder 73
hypogonadism 53
hypomania 40, 41

Improving Access to Psychological Therapies 103,
    106
inflexible coping behaviour 7–8
information
    patient-identifiable 94
    sources
        medication 101–2
        psychological therapies 106
        risk management 110
    technology 14
initial assessment 1–6
initial crisis management plan 27

injected drugs 21, 22, 45, 57, 98
insight 3
institutional care 15–18, 20, 23, 87–8, 91–3
integrated mental health care 23, 24, 26
integrative psychological therapy 105
intellect 3
intellectual disability 76–80
internalising disorders, children 73, 74
International Classification of Diseases 48, 49, 78
International Late Onset Schizophrenia Group 66
interview technique 2, 4, 10, 12
intramuscular route 21, 22, 45, 98
intravenous route 21, 22, 57

jiryan 83

laboratory tests 3, 69
lamotrigine 100
latah 83
late-onset paranoid disorders 66
law 91–5
  County Asylums Act (1845) 24
  Lunacy Act (1890) 24
  Lunatics Act 24
  Mental Capacity Act (2005) 3, 91, 92–3
  Mental Health Act 16, 19, 20, 25, 27, 48, 82, 83
    (1983) 48, 91–2
    (2007) 91, 93
  Mental Health (Patients in the community)
    Act (1995) 93
  Mental Treatment Act (1930) 24
  National Assistance Act (1948) 94
learning disability 74
Lesch–Nyhan syndrome 76
lithium 41, 42, 100
London, homelessness 87
long-term prediction 20, 109
lorazepam 21, 22
Lunacy Act (1890) 24
Lunatics Act 24

magistrates 92
major incidents 20–22
malignant social pathology 70
mania 40, 41, 47
mannerisms, distress 9
marijuana 56, 57, 58
marriage, arranged 84
MDMA 56, 57, 58
medical records 21, 25, 94, 110
medication 96–102
  alcohol abstinence 62–3
  anxiety disorders 29, 99–100
    obsessive–compulsive disorder 34
    older people 66
    panic disorder 30, 31
    post-traumatic stress disorder 33
  bipolar affective disorder 38, 41
  concordance with treatment 17, 101
  dementia 69–70, 71
  depression 36–7, 65, 96–7
  dosage/duration 97, 98, 100
  drug misuse 55–9
  intellectual disability 80
  interactions 57
  mood-stabilising 41, 42, 100
  personality disorders 51

preliminary physical tests 3
primary care 13
psychiatric disorder in physically-ill
    patients 17
  rapid tranquillisation 20–22
  schizophrenia 45–6, 97–9
  sexual dysfunction cause 53
  side effects 97, 99, 100
  social phobia 32
medium-term risks 109
memory clinics 70
Mental Capacity Act (2005) 3, 91, 92–3
Mental Health Act 16, 19, 20, 25, 27, 82, 83
    (1983) 48, 91–2
    (2007) 91, 93
Mental Health (Patients in the community)
    Act (1995) 93
Mental Health Review Tribunal 92, 93
mental hospitals 23
mental impairment 91
mentally disordered offenders/prisoners 93
mental state examination 3
Mental Treatment Act (1930) 24
methadone 58
3,4-methylenedioxymethamphetamine
    56, 57, 58
midazolam 21, 22
migration 83
MIND 5
mindfulness techniques 103, 104
Mini-Mental State Examination 68, 69
mirroring behaviour 9
mirtazapine 96
mixed affective states 41
moclobemide 37
modelling appropriate behaviour 9
monoamine oxidase inhibitors 36, 96
mood
  disorders
    see also depression
    bipolar 1, 38, 40–43, 79, 100
    children/adolescents 73, 74
    diagnostic hierarchies 4
    intellectual disability 78, 79
    physical illness-associated 16
    stabilising drugs 42, 51, 100
  mental state examination 3
morbidity 1, 11
mortality rates 5
multi-agency public protection
    arrangements 94
multidisciplinary approach 23, 24, 78, 88
multiethnic aspects 81–5
multisystems therapy 73

Nafsiyat Intercultural Therapy Centre 84
National Assistance Act (1948) 94
National Institute for Health and Clinical
    Excellence 13
  acetylcholinesterase inhibitors 69, 70
  anxiety disorders 28, 29, 30, 65
  attention deficit hyperactivity disorder 73, 74
  atypical antipsychotics 98
  depression 35
  psychological treatments 103, 105, 106
  self-harm guidelines 16
National Service Framework 24, 25, 64, 65, 74

National Survey of Psychiatric Morbidity in
    Great Britain 11
nearest relative 93
need 25, 26, 86
nefazodone 37
neuroleptic malignant syndrome 98
neurological assessment 3
neuroses
  anxiety 11–14, 17, 28–34, 65–6, 78–9, 88
  definition 4
NHS guidelines 10
NHS Plan 23, 24
no fixed address rotas 89
non-opioid drug withdrawal 58
non-statutory care provision 23, 62, 71
norms, cultural 81

obeah (curses) 82
obsessive–compulsive disorder 29, 33–4,
    74, 79
Office of National Statistics 28
olanzapine 21, 22, 41, 42, 97
older people 64–7
open/closed questions 2, 3
opioid misuse 56, 57, 58
oppositional defiant disorder 73
organic disease 4, 16, 20
outreach teams 24

pain management model 8
panic 8, 29, 30, 31, 32
paraldehyde 21, 22
paranoia 3, 45, 66
paraphilias 54
parenting/family 72, 73, 83–4, 93, 105
parkinsonian syndrome 99, 101
patient-held records 25
patient history 20, 77
patient-identifiable information 94
patient needs 25, 26, 86
perceptions 3
persecutory beliefs 3, 45, 66
personal accounts 5
  alcohol dependence 63
  anxiety disorders 34
  brain injury 10
  children/adolescents 75
  depression 39
  ethnic aspects 85
  hospital situation 18
  intellectual disability 80
  psychosexual problems 54
  schizophrenia 47
personality disorders 48–51
  aetiology 49
  diagnosis and assessment 48, 49–50
  epidemiology 49
  homelessness 87, 88
  hospital admission 50
  intellectual disability 78, 79
  medication 51
  prevalence 1
  psychological treatment 50–51
personality traits 4
pervasive developmental disorder 74
pharmacotherapy see medication
phobias 28, 29, 32, 74

physical aspects
  see also violence
  illness
    general hospital situation 15–18
    homelessness 88
    mental disorder-associated 12, 16–17
    older people 64–5
  physical tests 3
  sexual dysfunction 53
  stress 83
place of safety 92
plans 10, 19–20
police 21–2, 92, 94
population-based studies 11
possession by spirits 81, 82
postpartum depression 38
post-traumatic stress disorder 28, 29, 32–3
  children/adolescents 72
  homelessness 87
  intellectual disability 79
post-traumatic therapy 22
posture 9, 21
poverty 86–90
practical risk management 109–10
Prader–Willi syndrome 76
primary care
  child/adolescent mental health 72, 74
  counselling 104–5
  depression 35
  mental health problems in 11–14
  NICE guidelines 25
  reviews, proactive 14
  safety netting 14
  shared mental health care 24–5
  system development 14
  typologies of mental health problems 12
prison services 93, 94
private care 23
probation orders 94
professionals 21, 22, 108–9, 110
  attitude to homelessness 88
  carer support workers 24
  community mental health teams 23, 24,
    25, 26, 46
  crisis resolution/home treatment teams 24, 27
  gateway primary-secondary workers 25
  general practitioners 11–14, 24–5, 72, 74
  graduate primary care workers 25
  legal requirements 91–5
  multidisciplinary approach 23, 34, 78, 88, 94
  psychological treatments 103
  risk control 108–9, 110
  second opinion approved doctors 92
promethazine 22
psychiatric assessment 1–6, 78
Psychiatric Assessment Schedule for Adults with
    Developmental Disability 78
psychiatric emergencies 19–22, 41–2, 92
psychodynamic therapy 104, 105
psychologically-based physical syndromes 17, 18
psychological risk factors 20
psychological treatments 103–7
  anxiety disorders 29, 30
  basic hospital clinician skills 17
  choice 106
  depression in older people 65
  obsessive–compulsive disorder 34

organisations 107
panic disorder 31–2
personality disorders 50–51
post-traumatic stress disorder 33
primary care 13
schizophrenia 46
sexual dysfunction 54
social phobias 32
psychopathic disorders 91
psychoses 4, 11, 87–8
  see also psychotic disorders; schizophrenia
psychosexual disorders 52–4, 83
psychosocial impairment 73
psychosocial interventions 79, 80
psychotherapy 36
psychotic disorders 20, 37, 38, 55
  see also schizophrenia
puerperal psychosis 40

rapid tranquillisation 20–22
recognition 8–9, 12–13
recordkeeping 21, 25, 94, 110
recurrent depression 12
referral to specialists
  acute bipolar disorder states 41
  criteria 25
  dementia 70
  depression 36, 65
  intellectual disability 77
  personality disorders 49
  primary care function 13–14
  report components 4–5
reflecting patient distress 9
refugees 87
relapse prevention 42–3, 46
relationship problems 52
religion 82, 83
residential services 26
responsible clinician 93
restraint 21
Rethink 5, 102
review processes 14
risk 108–13
  Care Programme Approach 24
  child/adolescent mental health 72–3
  electroconvulsive therapy 38
  initial assessment 2–3
  management 108–10
  mental health emergencies 19–21
  primary care situation 13
  self-harm, hospital situation 16
  suicide 2, 15, 111
  violence 20
risperidone 22
Royal College of General Practitioners 10
Royal College of Psychiatrists 5

safety see risk
safety netting 14
St John's wort 97
schizophrenia 44–7
  antipsychotics 45–6, 97–9, 101
  cultural aspects 82, 83
  family intervention 105
  homelessness 86, 87
  intellectual disability 78–9
  older people 66

prevalence 1
Rethink 5, 102
violence risk 20, 110
school 72, 73, 74
seasonal affective disorder 38
secondary care
  see also referral to specialists
  bipolar disorder 41–2
  depression 36
  mental health services 23, 24–5
  NICE guidelines 25
  role 25
  teams 24–5, 26
second opinion approved doctors 92
sedation 97, 98
selective serotonin reuptake inhibitors 30, 96, 97
  depression 36, 37
  older people 65, 66
  social phobias 32
self-harm 1, 15–16, 39, 51, 77
self-help 30, 31, 33, 42–3
serotonin-noradrenaline reuptake
    inhibitors 36, 37
serotonin reuptake inhibitors 30, 96, 97
  depression 36, 37
  older people 65, 66
  social phobias 32
service models 80, 88–9, 90
service provision 23–7, 84, 87, 88, 89, 103
severe mental impairment 91
sexual dysfunction 17, 52–4
shared care 24–5
short-term prediction 20, 109
side effects 97, 98
  antidepressants 36, 37
  antiepileptic drugs 100
  antipsychotics 45, 101
  benzodiazepines 99
  lithium 100
simple schizophrenia 45
sleep disturbance 43
Smith–Magenis syndrome 76
social phobias 29, 32
social risk factors 20
social treatment 65, 70
sodium valproate 41, 42
somatic syndrome 36
somatisation 12, 17, 18, 82, 83
specialists see referral to specialists; secondary care
specific (isolated) phobias 32
speech 3
spirit possession 81, 82
staff see professionals
standardised mortality rate 5
stepped care model 13, 17
stereotyping 88
stigma 5, 11
stress 28, 83
substance misuse see drug misuse
suicide
  antidepressant risk 97
  depression 2, 13, 22, 39, 97, 111
  emergency situation 22
  lithium 100
  prevalence 1
  primary care questions 13
  risk 2, 15, 111

supervised discharge 93
susto 83
system development 14

tardive dyskinesia 99
team-based care 23, 24, 25, 26, 27, 46
teratogenicity 101
termination of interviews 10
terminology, troublesome 4
testamentary capacity 94
tests
    AUDIT 61
    laboratory tests 3
    risk assessment 109
third-wave approaches 103, 104
thoughts 3
    see also delusions; paranoia
trance-like states 82
TREC Collaborative Group 21
tricyclic antidepressants 30, 36, 37, 96
Tuke, William 23

two-phase surveys 11
typologies of problems 12

UK mental health service
        provision 23–7

valid consent 93
valproate 100–101
velocardiofacial syndrome 76
venlafaxine 37, 96
verbal expressions of distress 8, 9
violence
    emergencies 19–22
    NHS guidelines 10
    risk 20, 109–10, 111–12
    self-harm 1, 15–16, 39, 51, 77
vitamin B 62
volatile substance misuse 57, 58
voluntary organisations
    alcohol detoxification 62
    Alzheimer's disease 71

ethnic 84
    mental health service provision 23
    role 5
voting rights 94

watchful waiting 12, 13, 33
Williams syndrome 76
witchcraft 81, 82
withdrawal of non-opioid drugs 58
withdrawal syndrome 55, 56, 62
World Health Organization 1
    Alcohol Use Disorders Identification
        Test 61
    depression 35
    disability due to mental disorder 5
    ICD-10 classifications 37, 48, 49, 78
    study of mental disorder in general
        healthcare 11

Zito, Jonathan 24
zuclopenthixol acetate 21